# 2021 GLUTEN FREE BUYERS GUIDE

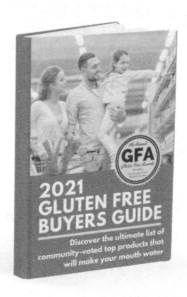

## JOSH SCHIEFFER

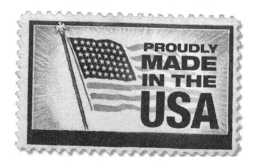

# Table of Contents

## Media - 152

## Other - 174

## Pasta, Sides, Soup & Sauces - 183

## Personalities - 197

# Introduction by Josh Schieffer

This happens to be our eighth Gluten Free Buyers Guide and our twelfth year hosting the Annual Gluten Free Awards. If you are not familiar with the book, I thought it would be best to explain what the book is and more importantly what it is not.

This book is much more than a list of great gluten free products to buy, we list some of the best locations and gluten free personalities. Being on a gluten free diet can be isolating in so many ways. With a heavy emphasis on celiac disease, we produce eye opening information gathered from polling our readers. Our goal is to ensure you do not feel so alone.

This book does not contain every single gluten free product available in every market. The gluten free industry has changed dramatically since we started in 2008. Virtually no regional grocery chains had private label gluten free products and now it is the norm with west coast chains like Safeway and east coast chains like Publix. We focus on brands with national distribution and national grocery chains. We do this so you have access to these products regardless of where you live. Oftentimes ordering online can save you money, time and widen your options dramatically.

You will not find every brand or product listed in this book on your local grocery shelves. It's a strange fact to some but often brands have to pay to sit on the shelves of most grocery stores. This is especially true for products that don't get purchased as often, like gluten free products. If you have a favorite product that your store doesn't carry, you can request that they stock it for a trial period. If it sells, more than likely they will keep it without the brand paying for the space. However, if a competing brand buys out the shelf space your product will more than likely disappear. This is the cold hard truth about the industry. Those of us who eat gluten free food to maintain a healthy lifestyle pay the price.

Gluten Free food is our medicine for a diagnosis we didn't want or ask for. Please use this guide to help make your gluten free lifestyle the best it can be.

Why do I tell you all of this? Those of us with restricted diets have limited options especially in rural parts of the country. I do not want your diet and the products you eat being dictated by what brands pay to sit on your local shelves. The product placement in your local store is not based on how great the product is and how well it tastes. If you want to have the best gluten free products in your pantry, more than likely you will need to travel to multiple stores and order online.

At the end of the day I want you to know that there are great gluten free products for you and your family. If you are new to the gluten free diet or just struggling to maintain the diet because of product availability or poor product quality, we published this book for you. Please read "Our Story" so you have a better understanding of why we have hundreds of product pictures and not just a list of a million random gluten free products.

This year we had 5,090 people take part in the voting process. The individual responses are all rolled up in the following pages. We added a few new gluten free award categories now totaling 62 and have organized the book in sections for easier navigation.

# HOW THE GLUTEN FREE AWARDS WORK

Presented by The Gluten Free Buyers Guide

## PRODUCT REGISTRATION

### Gluten Free Buyers Guide Registration

Each year brands register their products in The Gluten Free Buyers Guide. The guide consists of 60 gluten free categories ranging from gluten free bread to gluten free comfort food. Find more registration details at GlutenFreeBuyersGuide.com

## GLUTEN FREE BLOGGERS & INFLUENCERS

### Top bloggers & influences register products

We generate a list of 20-30 top gluten free bloggers and social media influencers. We ask them to register their favorite brands and products to be submitted into The Gluten Free Buyers Guide.

## COMMUNITY VOTE

### We ask the gluten free community to vote

Once we have the products registered for The Gluten Free Buyers Guide we create a voting ballot with those products listed in their respected categories. Nearly 10,000 people in the gluten free community vote for their favorites.

## PUBLISHING

### We publish The Gluten Free Buyers Guide

The Gluten Free Buyers Guide publishes all products that had been registered highlighting the top three GFA Award Winners in each category. The winners will have an image of their product so consumers can quickly identify those products while shopping.

# Our Story

*The story behind The Gluten Free Awards that very few people know*

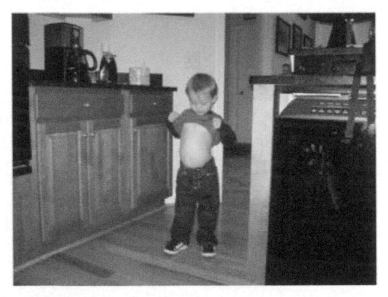

I remember it like it was yesterday when my four-year-old son Jacob, now fifteen, was playing in the kiddie pool with other kids that I assumed were his age based on their height. After asking all the surrounding kids what ages they were, I realized Jacob was significantly smaller than kids his own age. This prompted my wife and I to seek a professional opinion. After consulting with our family physician, she confirmed that Jacob had essentially stopped growing for an entire year without us realizing it. He was referred to Jeff Gordon's Children's Hospital in Charlotte North Carolina to discuss possible growth hormone therapy. The doctors there reviewed Jacob's case and requested a few blood tests based on some suspicions they had.

Our cell phone service at our house was terrible so when the doctor finally called with the blood results, my wife and I ran to the front of the driveway to hear the doctor clearly. With a sporadic signal, we heard "Jacob has celiac disease." We

4

looked at each other as tears ran down my wife's face. We huddled closer to the phone and asked, "what is celiac disease?". After getting a brief description mixed with crappy cell service and happy neighbors waving as they drove by, my wife and I embraced and wept. We were told to maintain his normal diet until we could have an endoscopy and biopsy for further confirmation. Once confirmed our next visit was to a registered dietitian for guidance.

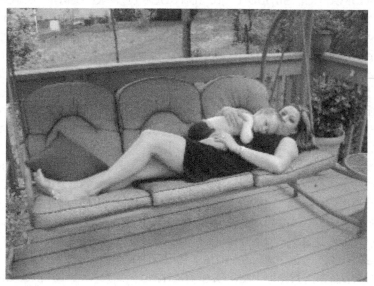

Jayme, my wife, made the appointment and called me with a weird request. "Will you meet me at the dietitian's house for a consultation?". I was confused when she said to go to her house. Jayme then explained that the dietician's daughter had celiac disease too and the best way to show the new lifestyle to patients would be to dive right in. I'll admit, it was a bit uncomfortable at first to be in a strangers' house looking at their personal items but looking back now, I wouldn't change it for the world. That encounter is ultimately the motivation behind The Gluten Free Awards and the associated Gluten Free Buyers Guide. We left her house with complete understanding of cross contamination, best practices and what products they personally liked and disliked. That visit was life changing and left us feeling confident as we made our way to the local health food store.

That first trip shopping took forever. Each label was read, and cross checked with our list of known gluten containing suspects. It was also shocking to see the bill when it was time to pay. We had replaced our entire pantry and fridge with all products that had the "Gluten Free" label. We both worked full-time and had decent paying jobs and it still set us back financially.

We looked for support groups locally and came across a "100% Gluten-Free Picnic" in Raleigh, which was two hours away from where we lived. This was our first time meeting other people with celiac disease and we were fortunate to have met some informative people that were willing to help with the hundreds of questions we had. We were introduced to a family whose son had been recently diagnosed with celiac disease as well. His condition was much worse than Jacobs and he was almost hospitalized before finally being diagnosed. They confided in us as we shared similar stories. There were two differences that would change my life forever. The first was the fact that they didn't have the same experience with a registered dietitian. Instead they were handed a two-page Xerox copy of "safe foods". Second, they didn't have the financial security to experiment with gluten free counterparts. Their first two months exposed to the gluten free lifestyle left them extremely depressed and broke.

On our way home from that picnic, Jayme and I felt compelled to help make a difference in some way. We were determined to help that family and others being diagnosed with this disease. Up until that day, we hadn't found a resource that gave unbiased opinions on gluten free products and services. Fast forward a few years and I too was diagnosed with celiac disease. That year, The Gluten Free Awards were born.

Originally our vision was to create a one-page website with a handful of categories organized by peoples' favorites. Since 2010 we have produced The Annual Gluten Free Awards (GFA) growing into sixty-two gluten free categories. After several requests, in 2014, we took the GFA results and published our first Gluten Free Buyers Guide. The annual guide is sold primarily in the United States however we continue to see increased global sales. Each year we have over 5,000 people vote for their favorite gluten free products and we now communicate to nearly 25,000 people weekly through our email list.

We want to thank those special people and organizations that brought us to where we are today:

Pat Fogarty MS, RD, LDN for allowing us to enter your home.

Jeff Gordon's Children's Hospital

Raleigh Celiac Support Groups

Dean Meisel, MD, FAAP for the excellent medical care he provides for our family.

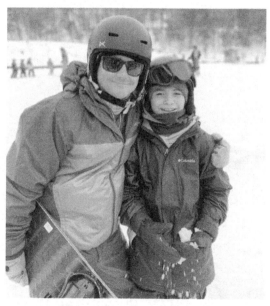

I hope you have learned something new from the story behind The Gluten Free Awards. Today, Jacob and I continue to live a healthy gluten free lifestyle.

# CELIAC SURVEY

We polled over 600 people with celiac disease
with the intent to make you feel not so alone.

## Should we be charged extra for a gluten free bun?

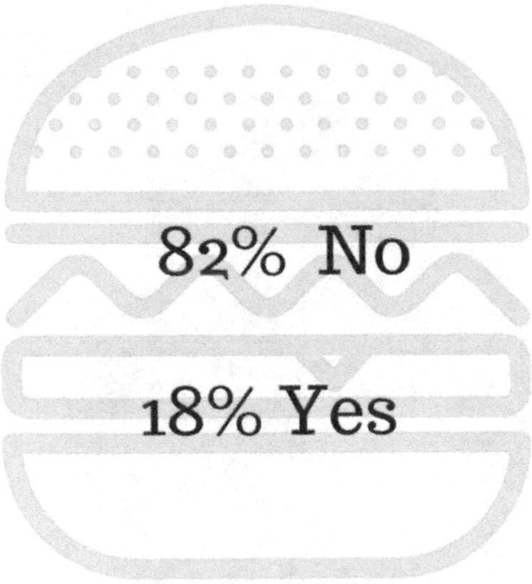

82% No

18% Yes

Presented by The 2021 Gluten Free Buyers Guide

## YOU'RE NOT ALONE

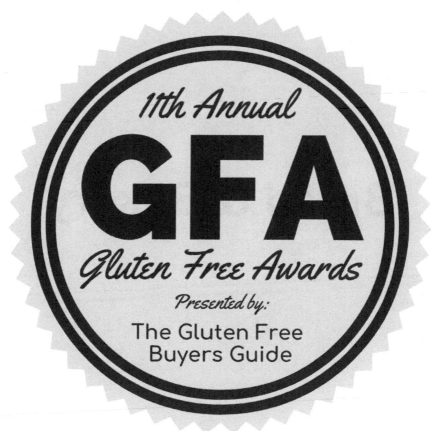

11th Annual

# GFA

Gluten Free Awards

Presented by:

The Gluten Free
Buyers Guide

# Bread & Bakery

# Bagels

## 11th Annual Gluten Free Awards

1st Place Winner:   Canyon Bakehouse Everything Bagel

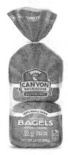

2nd Place Winner: ALDI-exclusive liveGfree Gluten Free Plain Bagels

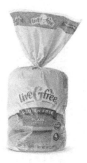

3rd Place Winner:   O'Doughs "Thins" Everything Bagels

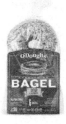

Runner Up: Schär Plain Bagel

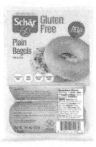

Other Great Products:

The Odd Bagel, Plain Bagel

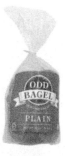

New Cascadia Traditional Sesame Bagels

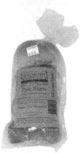

# CELIAC SURVEY

We polled over 600 people with celiac disease
with the intent to make you feel not so alone.

## How long have you had Celiac Disease?

### Average length: 16 years

### 9,494 combined years of experience

Presented by The 2021 Gluten Free Buyers Guide

## YOU'RE NOT ALONE

# Bread

## 11<sup>th</sup> Annual Gluten Free Awards

1<sup>st</sup> Place Winner:   Canyon Bakehouse 7-Grain

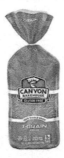

2<sup>nd</sup> Place Winner:   Canyon Bakehouse Heritage Honey Style White

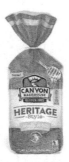

3<sup>rd</sup> Place Winner: Canyon Bakehouse Hawaiian Sweet Bread

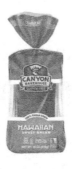

Runner Up:   O'Doughs "Thins" Original Sandwich

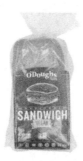

Other Great Products:

Mikey's English Muffins

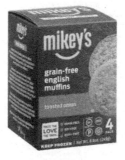

Lidl Gluten Free Cinnamon Raisin Bread

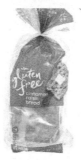

MYBREAD Original Flatbread Pitas

MYBREAD Baguettes

Lidl Gluten Free White Bread

MYBREAD Ancient Grain Flatbread Pitas

**Shop differentli.**®

# Gluten-free shouldn't taste like Gluten-free.

**Look for liveGfree®
products in store with
the liveGfree® logo.**

With over 70 Gluten-free items, made only with the most premium ingredients, ALDI makes their liveGfree® products taste just like they should.

# Gluten-free should taste like Italy.

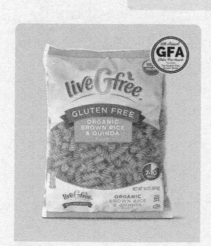

# Gluten-free
# should taste like it's right from the bakery.

# Gluten-free should taste like your favorite late-night snack.

# Bread Crumbs

## 11<sup>th</sup> Annual Gluten Free Awards

1<sup>st</sup> Place Winner:   Aleia's Gluten Free Italian Bread Crumbs

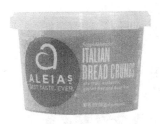

2<sup>nd</sup> Place Winner:   Aleia's Gluten Free Panko

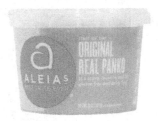

3<sup>rd</sup> Place Winner: Trader Joe's Rice Crumbs

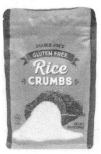

Runner Up:     Aleia's Coat & Crunch Extra Crispy

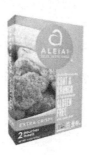

Other Great Products:

Michelle Farms Gluten Free Italian Bread Crumbs

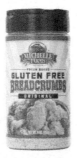

Appel Foods - Spicy Nut Crumbs

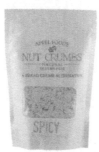

# Buns

## 11th Annual Gluten Free Awards

1st Place Winner: Canyon Bakehouse Stay Fresh Burger Buns

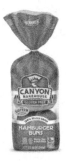

2nd Place Winner: Schär Hamburger Buns

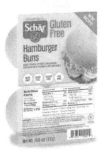

3rd Place Winner: O'Doughs Deluxe Hamburger Buns

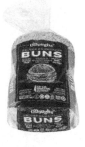

Runner Up:   Smart Bun - Gluten Free, Zero carbs of sugar, sesame, Hamburger Buns

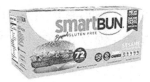

Other Great Products:

Little Northern Bakehouse Millet and Chia Gluten Free Hamburger Bun

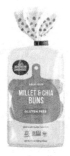

New Cascadia Traditional Gluten Free Hamburger Buns

Nuflours Gluten Free Bakery Hamburger Buns

# CELIAC SURVEY

We polled over 600 people with celiac disease
with the intent to make you feel not so alone.

## Have you helped anyone get diagnosed with Celiac Disease?

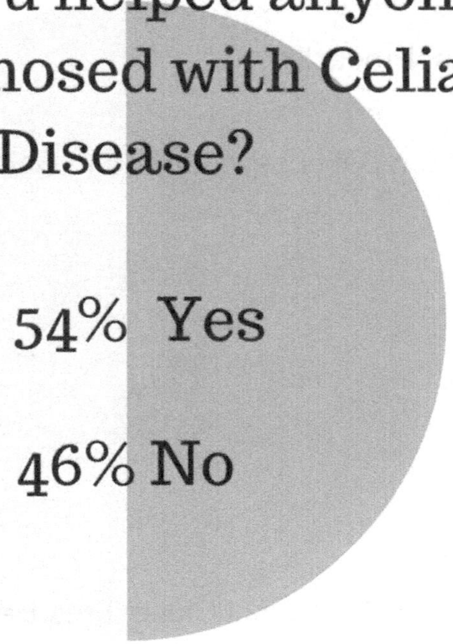

54% Yes

46% No

Presented by The 2021 Gluten Free Buyers Guide

## YOU'RE NOT ALONE

# Cookies

## 11th Annual Gluten Free Awards

1st Place Winner: Enjoy Life Foods - Soft Baked Snicker-doodle Cookies

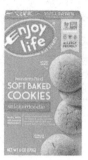

2nd Place Winner: Enjoy Life Foods Double Chocolate Brownie Soft Baked Cookies

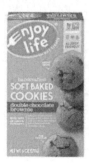

3rd Place Winner: Enjoy Life Foods - Crunchy Chocolate Chip Cookies

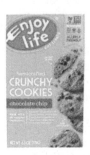

Runner Up: Brownie Brittle Gluten Free Dark Chocolate Sea Salt

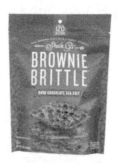

Other Great Products:

Brownie Brittle Gluten Free Chocolate Chip

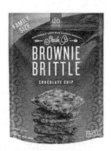

ALDI-exclusive Benton's Chocolatey Coconut Macaroons

MadeGood - Red Velvet Soft Baked Mini Cookies

ALDI-exclusive Benton's Coconut Macaroons

Goodman Gluten Free Chocolate Chip Cookies

Sweet Amsterdam Sea Salt & Caramel Stroopwafel

Goodman Gluten Free Brownie Cookie Bites

Goodman Gluten Free Chocolate Cookies with White Chips

Craize Guava Toasted Corn Crisps

Craize Coconut Toasted Corn Crisps

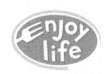

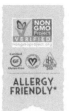

NON GMO Project VERIFIED nongmoproject.org

GF Certified Gluten-Free

ALLERGY FRIENDLY*

# SINCE 2001,
## *we have crafted*
### GLUTEN FREE & ALLERGY FRIENDLY
# SNACKS WITH
## *you in mind!*

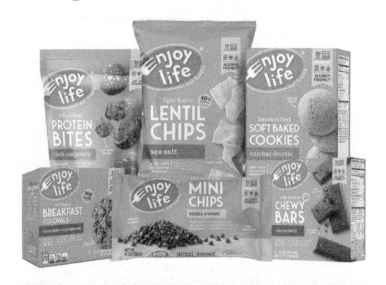

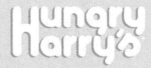
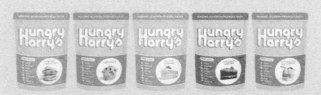
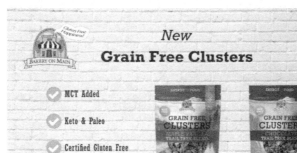

# Pizza Crust

## 11<sup>th</sup> Annual Gluten Free Awards

1st Place Winner:    GF Jules Pizza Crust Mix

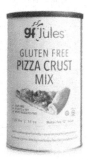

2nd Place Winner:    CAULIPOWER Cauliflower Crust

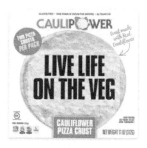

3rd Place Winner:    Pamela's Products Gluten Free Pizza Crust Mix

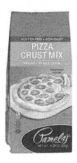

Runner Up: Wholly Gluten Free Pizza Dough Ball

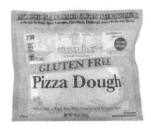

Other Great Products:

O'Doughs Original Flatbread

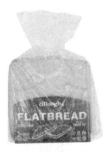

Zeia Foods Seasoned Crust

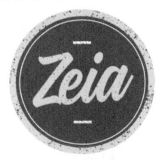

Stonewall Kitchen Gluten-free Herbed Pizza Crust Mix

Chebe - Gluten Free Pizza Crust Mix

# Rolls

## 11th Annual Gluten Free Awards

1st Place Winner:   Schar's Gluten Free Ciabatta Rolls

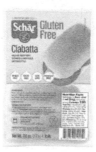

2nd Place Winner:   Udi's Gluten-free Classic French Dinner Rolls

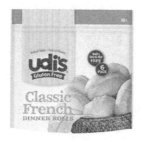

3rd Place Winner:   Against The Grain Original Rolls

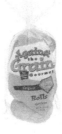

Runner Up:   MYBREAD Dinner Rolls

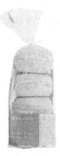

Other Great Products:

New Cascadia Traditionals Hoagie Rolls

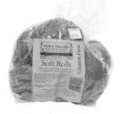

Something Sweet Without Wheat Dinner Rolls

# CELIAC SURVEY

We polled over 600 people with celiac disease
with the intent to make you feel not so alone.

Do you have anxiety when
eating out on a
gluten free diet?

78% Yes

22% No

Presented by The 2021 Gluten Free Buyers Guide

## YOU'RE NOT ALONE

# Tortilla or Wrap

## 11th Annual Gluten Free Awards

1st Place Winner:   Mission Gluten Free Corn Tortillas

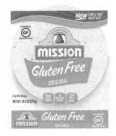

2nd Place Winner:   CAULIPOWER Cauliflower Tortillas

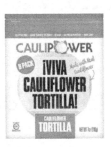

3rd Place Winner:   Siete Almond Flour Grain Free Tortillas

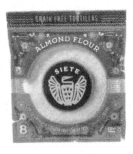

Runner Up:   Mikey's Tortillas

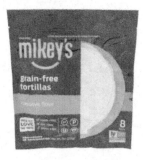

Other Great Products:

Parmesan Folios Cheese Wraps

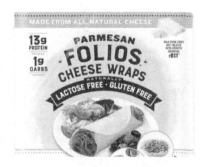

La Banderita Mini Taquito Corn Tortillas

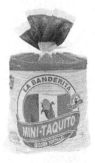

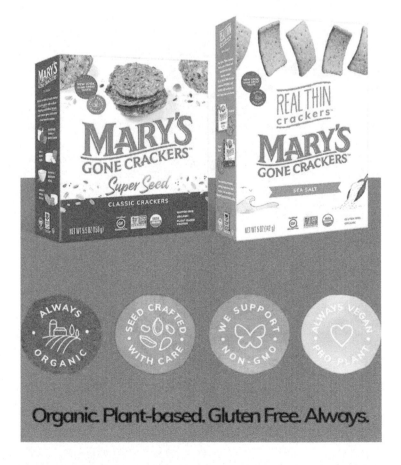

# Breakfast

# Breakfast On-The-Go

## 11ᵗʰ Annual Gluten Free Awards

1ˢᵗ Place Winner: Canyon Bakehouse Honey Whole Grain English Muffins

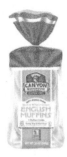

2ⁿᵈ Place Winner: Mikey's Egg, Ham and Cheese Breakfast Pockets

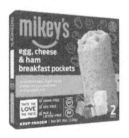

3ʳᵈ Place Winner: Enjoy Life Foods - Berry Medley Breakfast Ovals

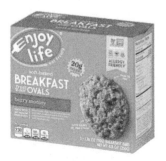

Runner Up:　siggi's Vanilla Plant-Based Yogurt

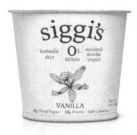

Other Great Products:

MadeGood - Cookies and Creme Granola Bars

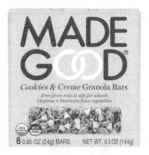

Bakery on Main Ancient Grain Instant Oatmeal

siggi's Mixed Berry Plant-Based Yogurt

Bakery on Main Organic Oats & Happiness Oatmeal Cups

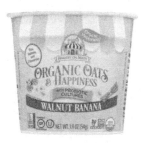

# Cold Cereals

## 11<sup>th</sup> Annual Gluten Free Awards

1<sup>st</sup> Place Winner:   Cinnamon Chex

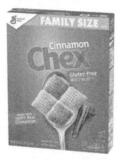

2<sup>nd</sup> Place Winner:   Bakery on Main Gluten-Free Granola

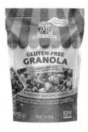

3<sup>rd</sup> Place Winner:   ALDI-exclusive Millville Crispy Rice Cereal

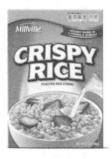

Runner Up:    Magic Spoon – Frosted

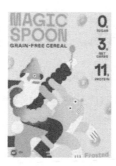

Other Great Products:

ALDI-exclusive Millville Rice Squares Cereal

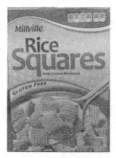

Love Grown Comet Crispies Cereal

ALDI-exclusive Millville Corn Squares Cereal

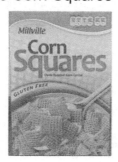

# CELIAC SURVEY

We polled over 600 people with celiac disease
with the intent to make you feel not so alone.

## Do you like to eat out or at home?

85% Home

15% Out

Presented by The 2021 Gluten Free Buyers Guide

## YOU'RE NOT ALONE

# Donuts

## 11th Annual Gluten Free Awards

1st Place Winner: Katz Gluten Free Glazed Chocolate Donuts

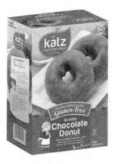

2nd Place Winner: ALDI-exclusive liveGfree Gluten Free Glazed Donuts

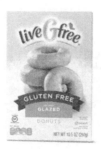

3rd Place Winner: ALDI-exclusive liveGfree Gluten Free Chocolate Donuts

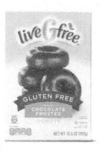

Runner Up:   Stonewall Kitchen Gluten Free Cinnamon Sugar Doughnut Mix

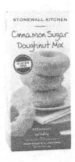

Other Great Products:

Freedom Old Fashioned Glazed Gluten Free Donuts

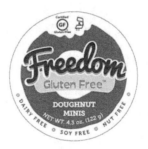

Diabetic Kitchen Cinnamon Keto Gluten Free Donut Mix

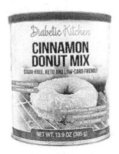

Measures of Joy Gluten Free Old-Fashioned Donut Mix

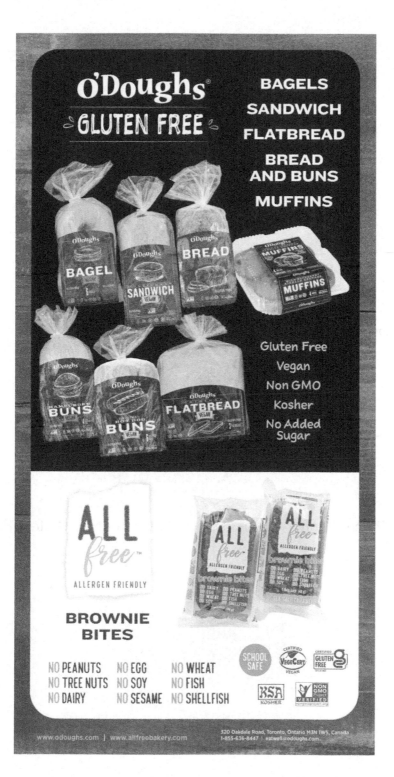

45

# Frozen Pancake & Waffle Brands

## 11th Annual Gluten Free Awards

1st Place Winner:    Van's Blueberry Waffles

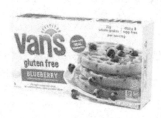

2nd Place Winner:    Trader Joe's Gluten Free Waffles

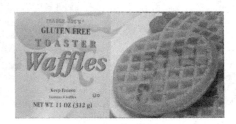

3rd Place Winner:    Nature's Path Homestyle Gluten Free Waffle

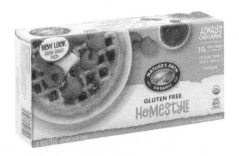

Runner Up:    Schär Golden Waffle (No need to freeze)

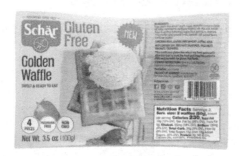

Other Great Products:

Birch Benders Paleo Frozen Waffles

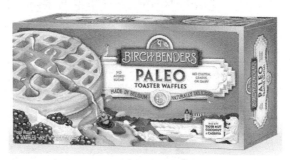

Lopaus Point Gluten Free Waffles

# Pancake and Waffle Mixes

## 11<sup>th</sup> Annual Gluten Free Awards

1<sup>st</sup> Place Winner:   gfJules Pancake & Waffle Mix

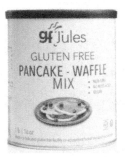

2<sup>nd</sup> Place Winner:   Birch Benders Gluten Free Pancake & Waffle Mix

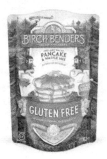

3<sup>rd</sup> Place Winner:   Better Batter Pancake and Biscuit Mix

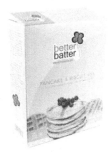

Runner Up:   Hungry Harry's Pancake and Waffle Mix

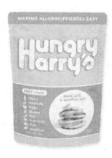

Other Great Products:

Whole Note Gluten Free Baking Mix, Buttermilk Pancake Mix

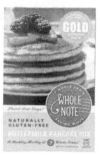

HighKey Snacks Keto Pancake & Waffle Mix

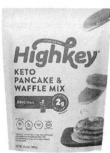

# CELIAC SURVEY

We polled over 600 people with celiac disease with the intent to make you feel not so alone.

## Opinion: How long will it take before they find a cure for Celiac Disease?

## Average: 38 More Years

Presented by The 2021 Gluten Free Buyers Guide

## YOU'RE NOT ALONE

# Cookies, Snacks & Candy

# Candy

## 11th Annual Gluten Free Awards

1st Place Winner:   Justin's Dark Chocolate Peanut Butter Crispy Cups

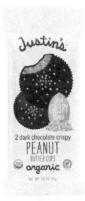

2nd Place Winner:   Enjoy Life Chocolate Bar - Ricemilk Crunch

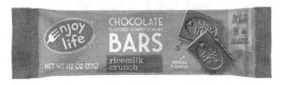

3rd Place Winner:   Schär Twin Bar

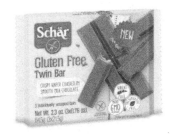

Runner Up:   No Whey! Milkless Crunchy

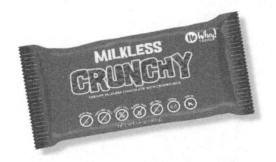

Other Great Products:

No Whey! Peppermint No No's

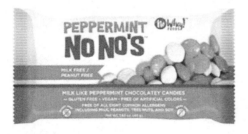

Torie & Howard   Chewie Fruities Sour Berry

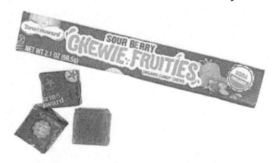

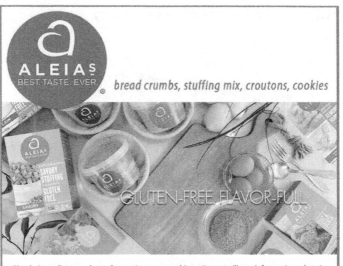
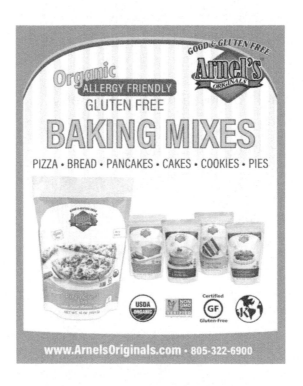

# Chips

## 11th Annual Gluten Free Awards

1st Place Winner:   Late July Nacho Chipotle Tortilla Chips

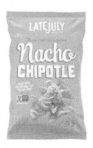

2nd Place Winner:   ALDI-exclusive Simply Nature Organic Yellow Corn Tortilla Chips

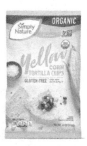

3rd Place Winner:   Siete Foods Ranch Grain Free Tortilla Chips

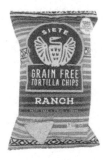

Runner Up:    Enjoy Life Foods - Sea Salt Lentil Chips

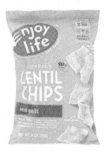

Other Great Products:

ALDI-exclusive Simply Nature Exotic Vegetable Chips

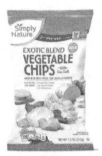

ALDI-exclusive Simply Nature White Bean Chips

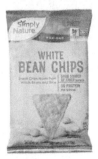

# Crackers

## 11th Annual Gluten Free Awards

1st Place Winner:   Schär Multigrain Table Cracker

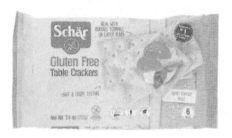

2nd Place Winner:   Simple Mills Veggie Pita Crackers

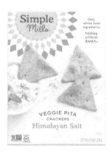

3rd Place Winner:   Mary's Gone Crackers Original

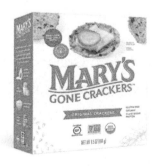

Runner Up:    Mary's Gone Crackers Super Seed Classic

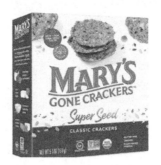

Other Great Products:

Mary's Gone Crackers REAL Thin Crackers Sea Salt

ALDI-exclusive Simply Nature Cheddar Cauliflower Crackers

ALDI-exclusive Simply Nature Sea Salt Cauliflower Crackers

Pipcorn Heirloom Everything Bagel Crackers

ALDI-exclusive Savoritz Jalapeno Parmesan Crisps

San-J Black Sesame Rice Crackers

Cult Crackers Classic Seed Crackers

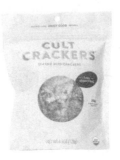

Craize Sweet Toasted Corn Crisps

Craize Seeded Toasted Corn Crisps

Craize Plantain Toasted Corn Crisps

# CELIAC SURVEY

We polled over 600 people with celiac disease with the intent to make you feel not so alone.

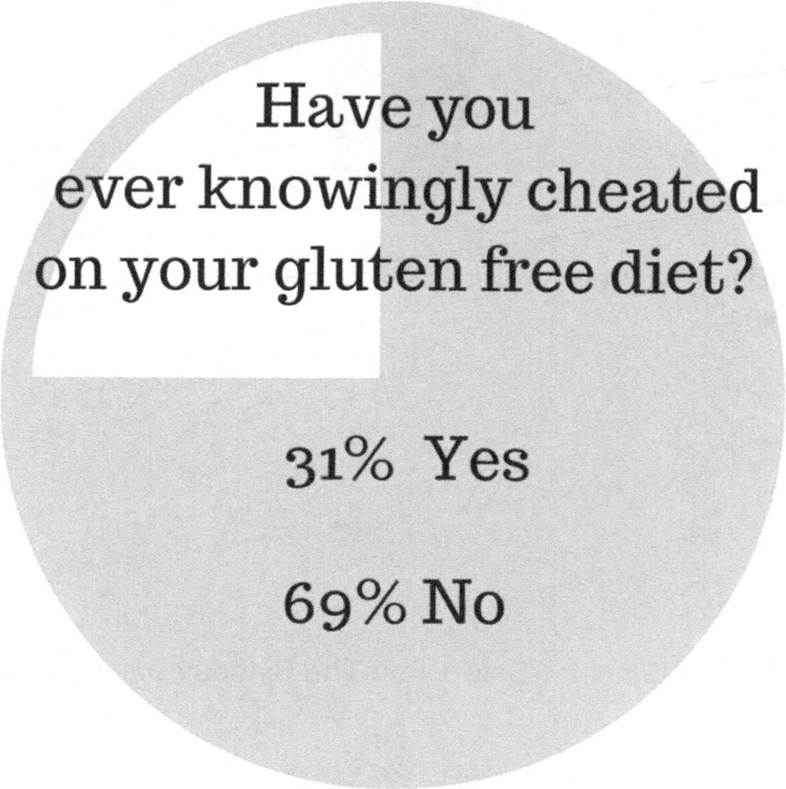

Have you
ever knowingly cheated
on your gluten free diet?

31% Yes

69% No

Presented by The 2021 Gluten Free Buyers Guide

## YOU'RE NOT ALONE

# Granola

## 11th Annual Gluten Free Awards

1st Place Winner:  Bakery on Main Bunches of Crunches Grain-ola

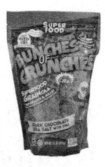

2nd Place Winner:  Purely Elizabeth Ancient Grain Granola, Original

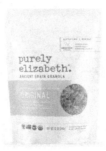

3rd Place Winner:  Safe + Fair The Birthday Cake Bundle

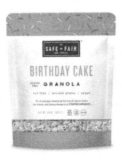

Runner Up:   Erin Baker's Homestyle Granola, Vanilla Almond Quinoa, Gluten-Free

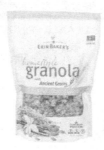

Other Great Products:

Autumn's Gold Grain Free Granola

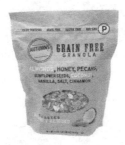

Ms. P's Gluten Free Granola

Goodness Grainless Granola Chocolate Cardamom

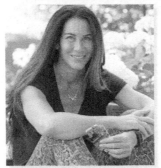
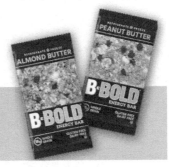
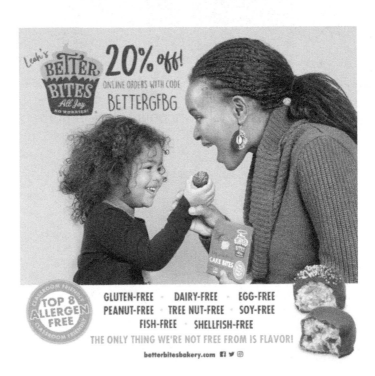

# Jerky

## 11th Annual Gluten Free Awards

1st Place Winner:   The New Primal Sea Salt Beef Thins

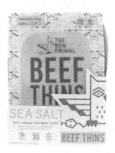

2nd Place Winner:   ALDI-exclusive Simms Aloha Teriyaki Artisan Jerky

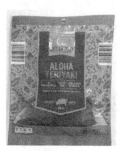

3rd Place Winner:   Real Hot & Spicy Beef Stick

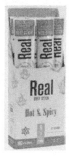

Runner Up:    Baja Jerky Lime & Serrano Pepper Beef Jerky

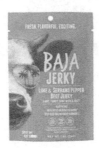

Other Great Products:

ALDI-exclusive Simms Spicy Garlic Artisan Jerky

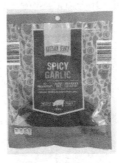

ALDI-exclusive Simms Chili Lime Artisan Jerky

# Munchies

## 11th Annual Gluten Free Awards

1st Place Winner:   Enjoy Life Foods - Dark Raspberry Protein Bites

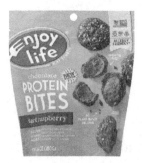

2nd Place Winner:   ALDI-exclusive Simply Nature Organic White Cheddar Puffs

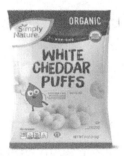

3rd Place Winner:   ALDI-exclusive Clancy's White Cheddar Cheese Popcorn

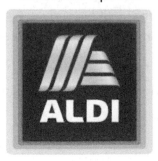

Runner Up:   ALDI-exclusive Clancy's Veggie Straws

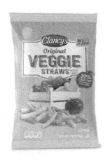

Other Great Products:

FatBoy® Gluten-Free Ice Cream Sandwich

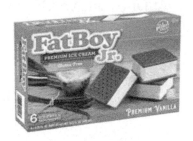

Pipcorn Jalapeño Cheddar Cheese Balls

GOODTO GO™ Cinnamon Pecan Soft Baked Bar

GOODTO GO™ Strawberry Macadamia Nut Soft Baked Bar

Real Garlic & Herb Beef Stick

Setton Farms Garlic Onion Seasoned Pistachio Kernels

Setton Farms Salt & Pepper Seasoned Pistachio Kernels

Setton Farms Jalapeno Seasoned Pistachio Kernels

# CELIAC SURVEY

We polled over 600 people with celiac disease with the intent to make you feel not so alone.

## After consuming gluten, do you have symptoms?

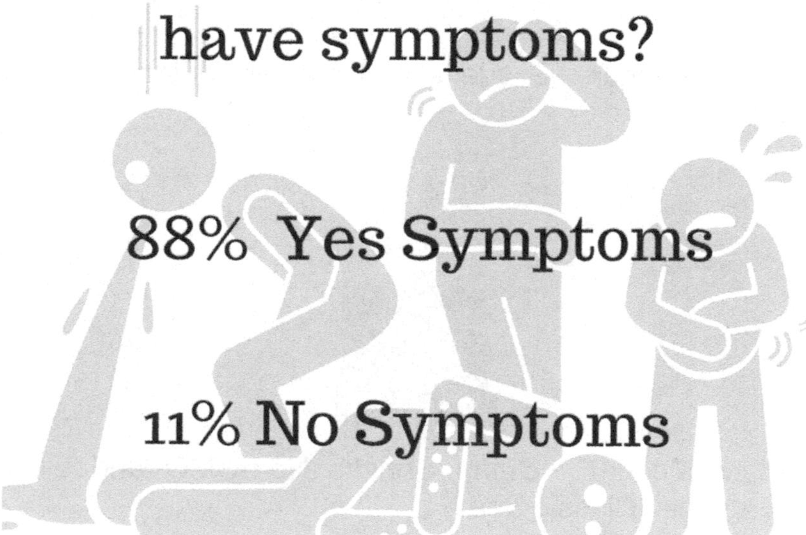

88%  Yes Symptoms

11% No Symptoms

Presented by The 2021 Gluten Free Buyers Guide

## YOU'RE NOT ALONE

# Pretzels

## 11th Annual Gluten Free Awards

1st Place Winner:   Snyder's of Hanover Gluten Free Pretzel Sticks

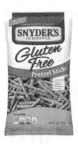

2nd Place Winner:   Snyder's of Hanover Gluten Free Mini Pretzels

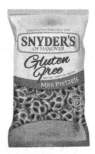

3rd Place Winner:   Quinn Snacks Non-GMO and Gluten Free Pretzels, Classic Sea

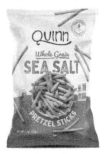

Runner Up:   Savor Street Grain Free Pretzel Twists - Gluten Free - Paleo Friendly

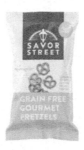

Other Great Products:

Lidl Gluten Free Mini Pretzel Twists

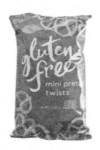

FitJoy Grain Free Pretzels, Gluten Free

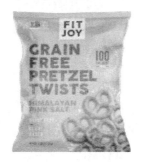

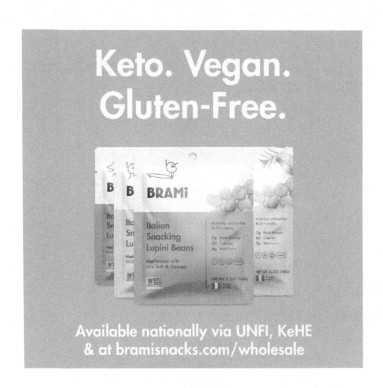
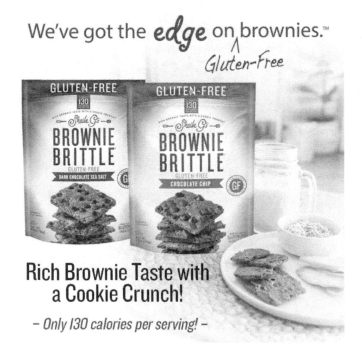

# Snack Bars

## 11th Annual Gluten Free Awards

1st Place Winner:  Enjoy Life Foods Cocoa Loco Bars

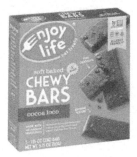

2nd Place Winner:  Fody Dark Chocolate Nuts & Sea Salt

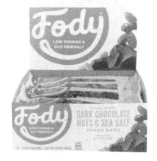

3rd Place Winner:  GOODTO GO™ Blueberry Cashew Soft Baked Bar

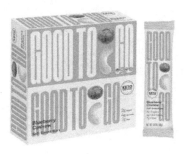

# Runner Up:   GOODTO GO™ Chocolate Mint Soft Baked Bar

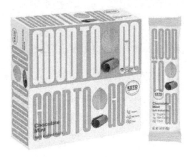

## Other Great Products:

BeBOLD Almond Butter Bar

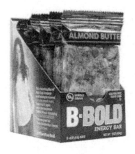

Fody Almond Coconut

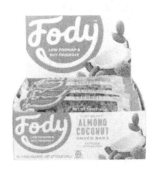

# Dessert

# Ice Cream Cones

## 11th Annual Gluten Free Awards

1st Place Winner:   Joy Gluten-Free Sugar Ice Cream Cones

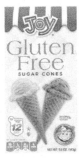

2nd Place Winner:   Joy Gluten-Free Ice Cream Cones Cake Cups

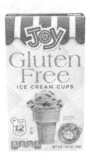

3rd Place Winner:   Jolly Llama Dairy-Free Gluten-Free Caramel Chocolate Chip Cone

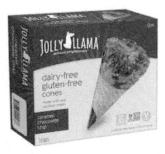

Runner Up:   Sprouts Coconut Cones

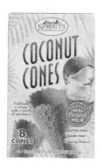

Other Great Products:

Edward & Sons Trading Co Cones, Sugar, Gluten Free

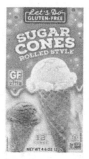

Barkat Gluten Free Waffle Ice Cream Cones

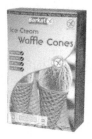

# CELIAC SURVEY

We polled over 600 people with celiac disease
with the intent to make you feel not so alone.

## Do you
## have other family with
## Celiac Disease?

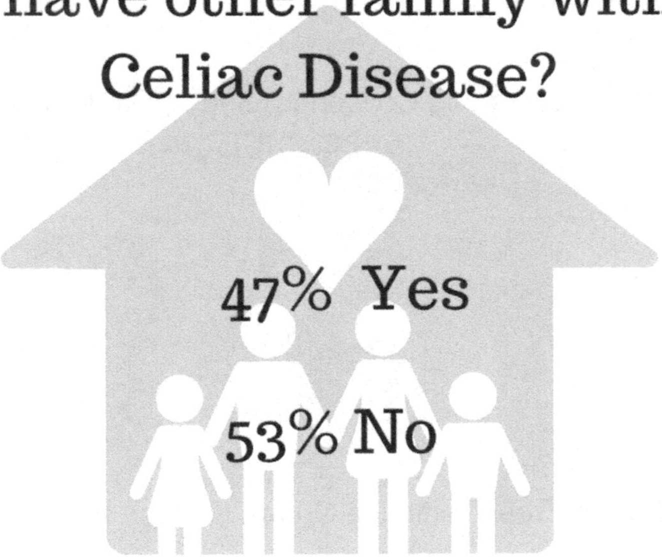

47% Yes

53% No

Presented by The 2021 Gluten Free Buyers Guide

## YOU'RE NOT ALONE

# Pie Crust

## 11th Annual Gluten Free Awards

1st Place Winner: Wholly Wholesome Gluten Free 9" Pie Shells

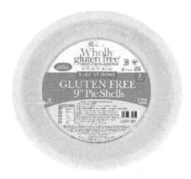

2nd Place Winner: Trader Joe's Frozen Pie Crust

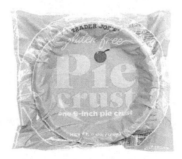

3rd Place Winner: Midel Graham Cracker Crust

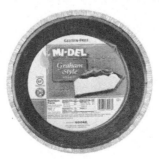

Runner Up:    Cup4cup Gluten-Free Pie Crust Mix

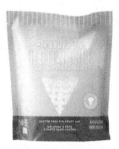

Other Great Products:

Maine Pie Co Frozen Pie Crust

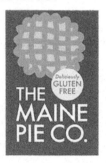

Williams Sonoma Gluten-Free Pie Crust Mix

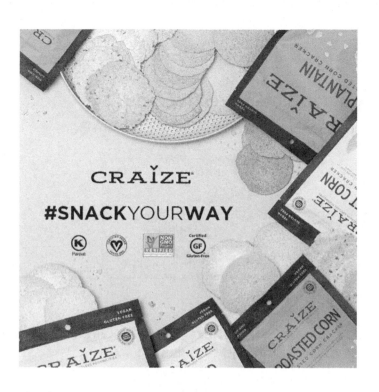

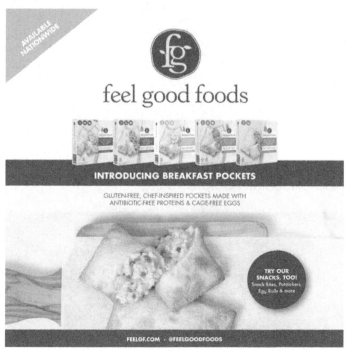

# Ready Made Desserts

## 11th Annual Gluten Free Awards

1st Place Winner:   Coconut Bliss Ice Cream Bars

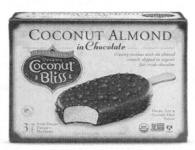

2nd Place Winner:   ALDI-exclusive liveGfree Gluten Free Soft Baked Snickerdoodle Cookies

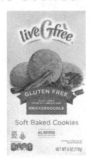

3rd Place Winner:   ALDI-exclusive liveGfree Gluten Free Soft Baked Chocolate Chip Cookies

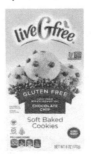

Runner Up:   Hail Merry Lemon Tart

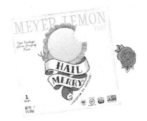

Other Great Products:

Better Bites BIRTHDAY DŌ BITES

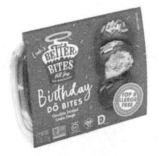

FatBoy® Gluten-Free Ice Cream Cone

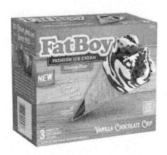

ALLfree Caramel Sea Salt Brownie Bites

Doodle Eats Strawberry Doodle Pie

# Beverages

# Beer

## 11<sup>th</sup> Annual Gluten Free Awards

1<sup>st</sup> Place Winner:   Glutenberg

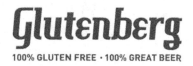

2<sup>nd</sup> Place Winner:   Ghostfish Brewing

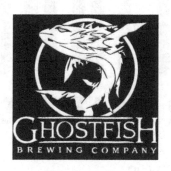

3<sup>rd</sup> Place Winner: New Grist

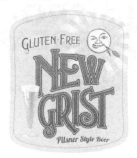

Runner Up:   Bards

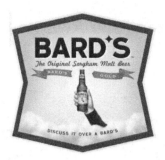

Other Great Products:

Holidaily Brewing

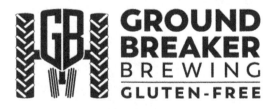

Ground Breaker Brewing

GROUND
BREAKER
BREWING
GLUTEN-FREE

# CELIAC SURVEY

We polled over 600 people with celiac disease
with the intent to make you feel not so alone.

## Do you drink gluten removed beer or stick to gluten free beers?

84% Gluten Free Only

6% Gluten Removed

10% Both

Presented by The 2021 Gluten Free Buyers Guide

## YOU'RE NOT ALONE

# Hard Cider

## 11th Annual Gluten Free Awards

1st Place Winner:   Angry Orchard Stone Dry Hard Cider

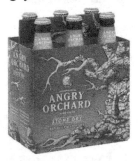

2nd Place Winner:   ALDI-exclusive Wicked Grove Hard Cider

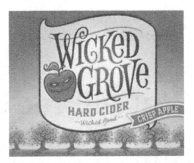

3rd Place Winner:   Austin Eastciders Blood Orange Cider

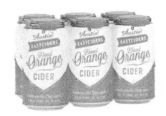

Runner Up:   California Cider Company ACE Cider Joker

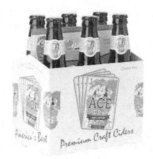

Other Great Products:

2 Towns Ciderhouse Easy Squeezy Raspberry Lemonade Cider

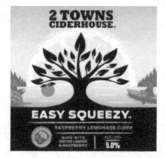

Blake's Cider El Chavo Mango & Habanero

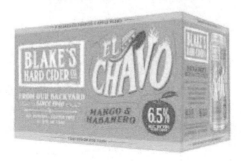

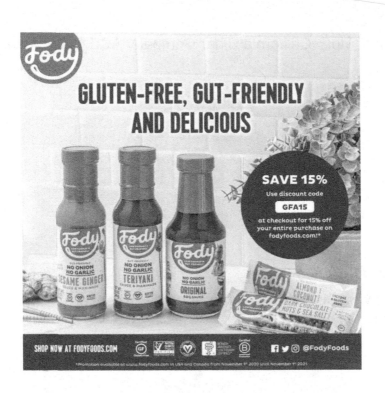

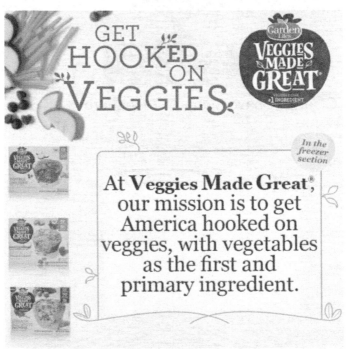

# Hard Seltzer

## 11th Annual Gluten Free Awards

1st Place Winner:   White Claw Mango Hard Seltzer

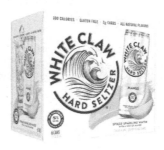

2nd Place Winner:   Truly Strawberry Lemonade Hard Seltzer

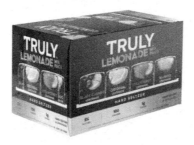

3rd Place Winner:   White Claw Watermelon

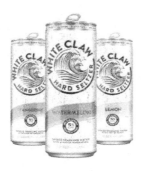

Runner Up:   Truly Raspberry Lime Hard Seltzer

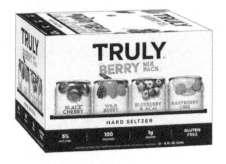

Other Great Products:

ALDI-exclusive Vista Bay Black Cherry Hard Seltzer

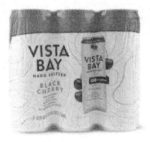

ALDI-exclusive Vista Bay Coconut Mango Hard Seltzer

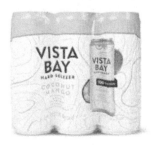

# Dry Mixes

# Bread Mixes

## 11th Annual Gluten Free Awards

1st Place Winner:   gfJules Bread Mix

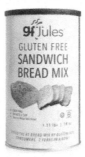

2nd Place Winner:   Bob's Red Mill Gluten Free Hearty Whole Grain Bread Mix

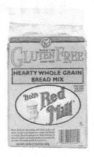

3rd Place Winner:   Pamela's Products Gluten-free Bread Mix

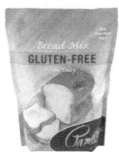

Runner Up:   Chebe Gluten Free Original Cheese Bread Mix

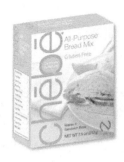

Other Great Products:

Big River Grains Bread Mix

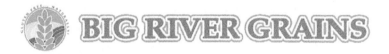

Good Dee's Multi-Purpose Gluten Free Bread Mix

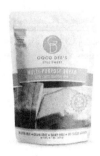

# CELIAC SURVEY

We polled over 600 people with celiac disease
with the intent to make you feel not so alone.

## At work, are you the only one with Celiac Disease?

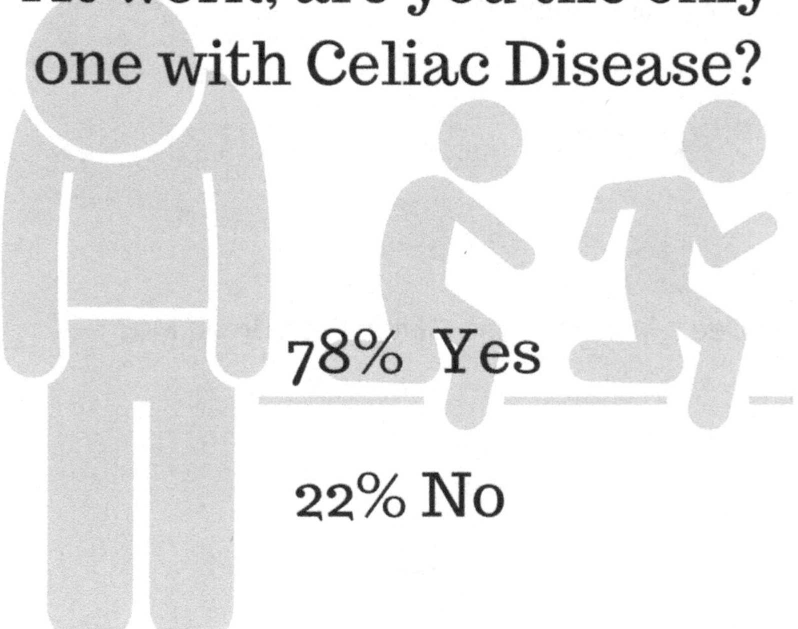

78% Yes

22% No

Presented by The 2021 Gluten Free Buyers Guide

## YOU'RE NOT ALONE

# Brownie Mixes

## 11th Annual Gluten Free Awards

1st Place Winner:  King Arthur Flour Gluten Free Brownie Mix

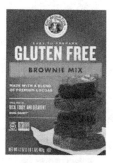

2nd Place Winner:  Pamela's Products Gluten Free Chocolate Brownie Mix

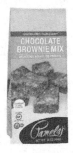

3rd Place Winner: Trader Joe's Gluten Free Chocolate Chip Brownie Mix

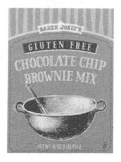

Runner Up: Better Batter Fudge Brownie Mix

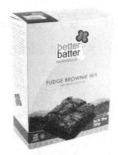

Other Great Products:

Keto Brownie Chocolate Chip Double Fudge Gluten Free Brownie Baking Mix

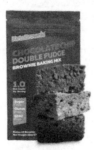

Renewal Mill Dark Chocolate Gluten Free Brownie Mix

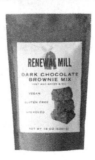

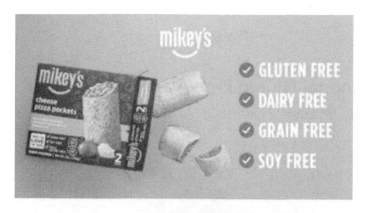

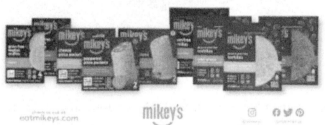

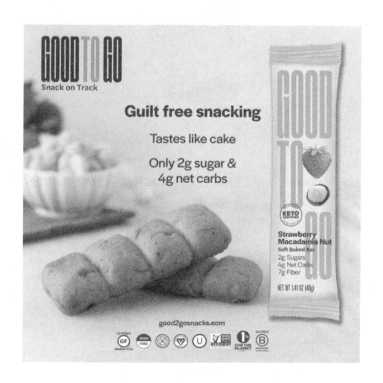

# Cake Mixes

## 11th Annual Gluten Free Awards

1st Place Winner:   Namaste Yellow Cake Mix

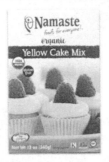

2nd Place Winner:   ALDI-exclusive liveGfree Gluten Free Angel Food Cake Mix

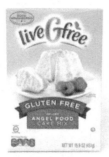

3rd Place Winner:   ALDI-exclusive liveGfree Gluten Free Lemon Cake Mix

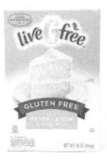

Runner Up:   Better Batter Chocolate Cake Mix

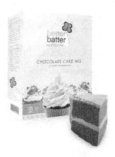

Other Great Products:

Better Batter Yellow Cake Mix

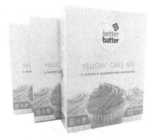

Hungry Harry's Chocolate Cake

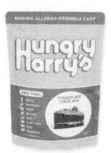

ALDI-exclusive liveGfree Gluten Free Key Lime Cake Mix

Hungry Harry's Yellow Cake

# Cookie Mixes

## 11<sup>th</sup> Annual Gluten Free Awards

1<sup>st</sup> Place Winner:   gfJules Cookie Mix

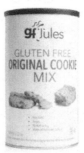

2<sup>nd</sup> Place Winner:   Sweet Loren's Chocolate Chunk Cookie Dough

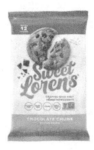

3<sup>rd</sup> Place Winner:   Hodgson Mill Gluten Free Cookie Mix

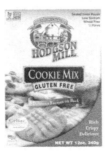

Runner Up:   Meli's Monster Gluten Free Cookies (Original)

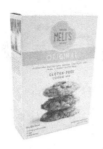

Other Great Products:

Good Dee's Butter Pecan Cookie Mix

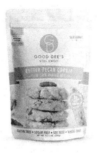

Ella Bella Chocolate Chip Cookie Mix

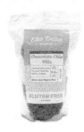

# CELIAC SURVEY

We polled over 600 people with celiac disease with the intent to make you feel not so alone.

## Do you have a dedicated gluten free toaster in your kitchen?

72% Yes

28% No

Presented by The 2021 Gluten Free Buyers Guide

## YOU'RE NOT ALONE

# Cornbread Mixes

## 11th Annual Gluten Free Awards

1st Place Winner:   gfJules Cornbread Mix

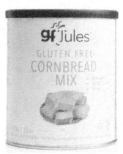

2nd Place Winner:   Stonewall Kitchen Gluten Free Corn-bread Mix

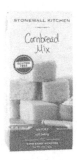

3rd Place Winner:   Really Great Food Company – Gluten Free Cornbread Muffin Mix

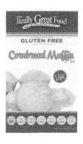

Runner Up: Good Dee's Corn Bread Baking Mix - Grain Free, Sugar Free, Gluten Free, Wheat Free, and Low Carb

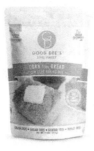

Other Great Products:

XO Baking Co. Corn Bread Mix

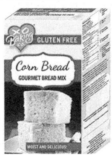

Miss Jones Baking Keto Not Cornbread Muffin Mix

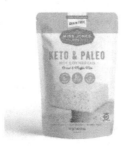

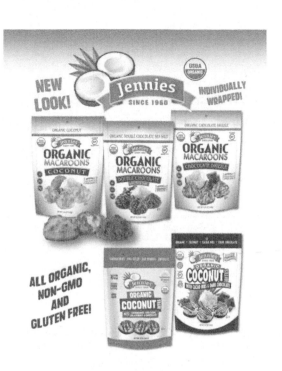

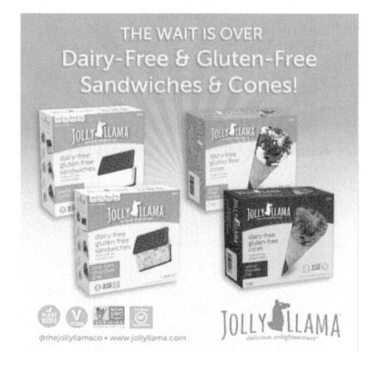

# Flours

## 11th Annual Gluten Free Awards

1st Place Winner:   gfJules All Purpose Gluten Free Flour

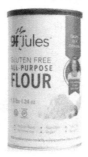

2nd Place Winner:   Cup 4 Cup™ Gluten Free Flour Blend

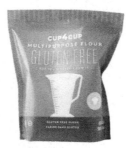

3rd Place Winner:   Trader Joe's Gluten Free All Purpose Flour

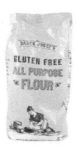

Runner Up:   Better Batter All Purpose Flour Mix

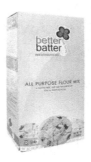

Other Great Products:

Better Batter Artisan Baker's Blend (Gum Free Flour Mix)

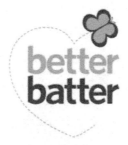

Hungry Harry's All Purpose Flour

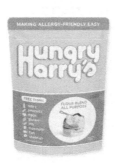

# Muffin Mixes

## 11th Annual Gluten Free Awards

1st Place Winner:   gfJules Muffin Mix

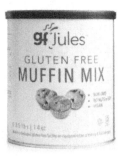

2nd Place Winner:   Namaste Foods Gluten Free Muffin Mix

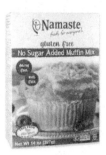

3rd Place Winner:   Hungry Harry's Muffin Mix

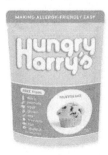

Runner Up: Vitacost Blueberry Muffin Mix - Non-GMO and Gluten Free

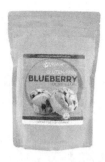

Other Great Products:

Keto and Co Banana Caramel Keto Muffin Mix

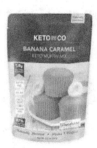

Good Dee's Lemon Muffin Mix - Gluten Free

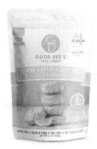

# CELIAC SURVEY

We polled over 600 people with celiac disease with the intent to make you feel not so alone.

Do you
try to keep your diagnosis
a secret or do you share
your story?

58%  Share
42%  It depends
0% Keep it secret

Presented by The 2021 Gluten Free Buyers Guide

## YOU'RE NOT ALONE

# Frozen Foods

# Frozen Food

## 11th Annual Gluten Free Awards

1st Place Winner:    CAULIPOWER Cauliflower Crust Pizza

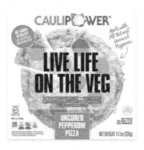

2nd Place Winner:    Mikey's Pepperoni Pizza Pockets

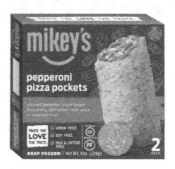

3rd Place Winner: Wholly Gluten Free Pizza Dough Ball

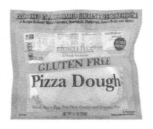

Runner Up:   Veggies Made Great Double Chocolate Muffin

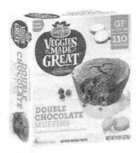

Other Great Products:

ALDI-exclusive Whole & Simple Mediterranean Chicken Quinoa Bowls

ALDI-exclusive Whole & Simple Southwest Chicken Quinoa Bowls

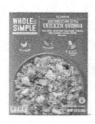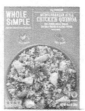

Veggies Made Great Spinach Egg White Frittata

Veggies Made Great Superfood Veggie Cakes

I MADE THE
**PERFECT**
COMBINATION
MORE PERFECTER

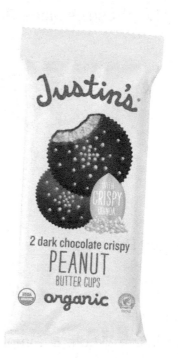

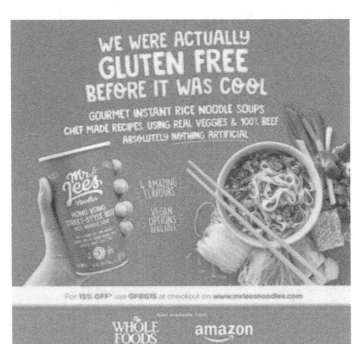

# Frozen Meals

## 11th Annual Gluten Free Awards

1st Place Winner:   Amy's Gluten Free Mac and Cheese

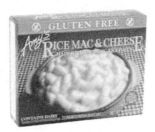

2nd Place Winner:   Applegate Gluten Free Chicken Tenders

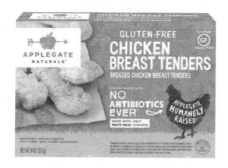

3rd Place Winner:   CAULIPOWER BAKED (never fried) Chicken Tenders

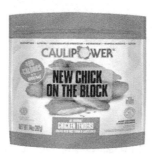

Runner Up:  ALDI-exclusive liveGfree Gluten Free Buffalo Chicken Stuffed Sandwich

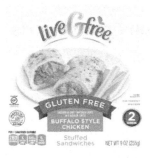

Other Great Products:

ALDI-exclusive liveGfree Gluten Free Spinach, Artichoke and Kale Stuffed Sandwich

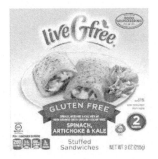

ALDI-exclusive liveGfree Gluten Free Southwest Veggie Stuffed Sandwich

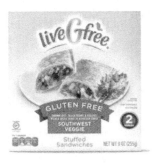

Rollin Greens Organic Basil & Garlic Ancient Grain Tots

# Frozen Pizza Brands

## 11<sup>th</sup> Annual Gluten Free Awards

1st Place Winner:   Freschetta

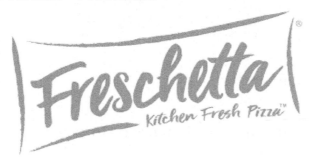

2nd Place Winner:   CAULIPOWER Cauliflower Crust Pizza

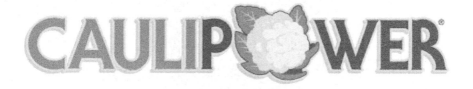

3rd Place Winner:   Against the Grain Gourmet

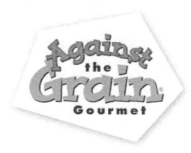

Runner Up: Sonoma Flatbreads

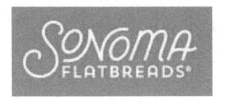

Other Great Products:

ALDI-exclusive liveGfree Gluten Free Pizzas

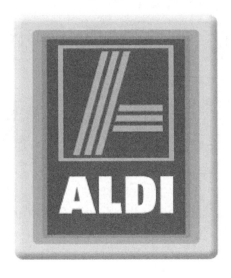

# CELIAC SURVEY

We polled over 600 people with celiac disease
with the intent to make you feel not so alone.

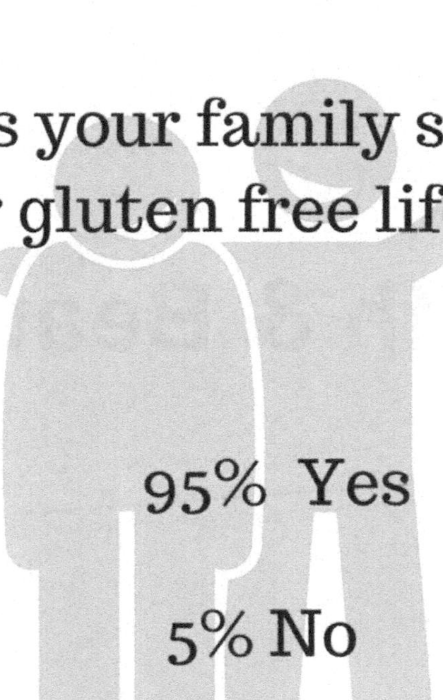

Does your family support
your gluten free lifestyle?

95% Yes

5% No

Presented by The 2021 Gluten Free Buyers Guide

## YOU'RE NOT ALONE

# Health & Beauty

# Cosmetic Brands

## 11th Annual Gluten Free Awards

1st Place Winner:   Tarte

tarte
high-performance naturals™

2nd Place Winner:   Red Apple Lipstick

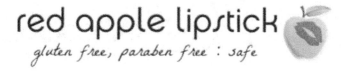

red apple lipstick
gluten free, paraben free : safe

3rd Place Winner:   DERMA E

DERMA·E

Runner Up: Afterglow

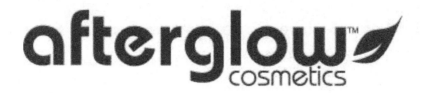

Other Great Products:

Au Naturale

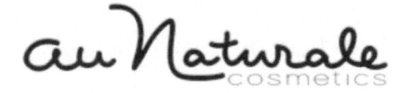

Kiss Freely

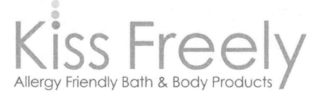

ILIA Beauty

Gabriel Cosmetics

Bellaphoria Organic Cosmetics

Lily Lolo

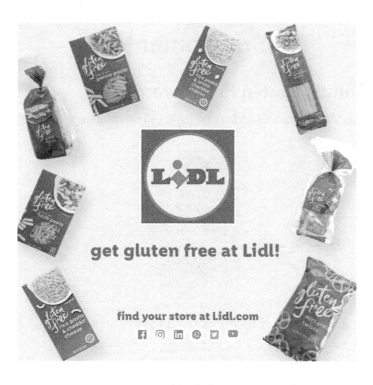
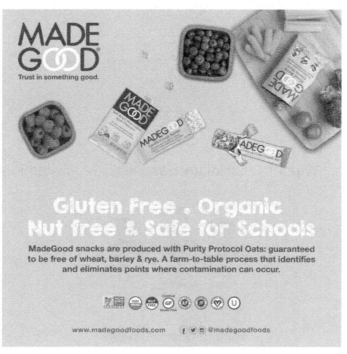

# Supplements

## 11th Annual Gluten Free Awards

1st Place Winner: Garden of Life Gluten Free Support

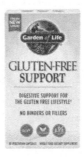

2nd Place Winner: MegaFood – Daily

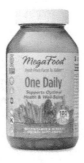

3rd Place Winner: ChildLife Essentials Multivitamin & Mineral

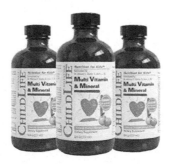

Runner Up:   Organifi Green Juice

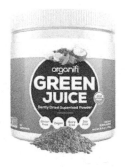

Other Great Products:

Standard Process Whole Food Fiber

Jarrow - Organic Plant Protein Salted Caramel

ChildLife Essentials Liquid Vit. C

# Locations

# College Campuses

## 11th Annual Gluten Free Awards

1st Place Winner:   UNIVERSITY OF CALIFORNIA, LOS ANGELES

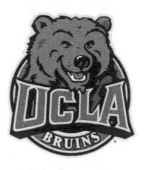

2nd Place Winner:   UNIVERSITY OF NOTRE DAME

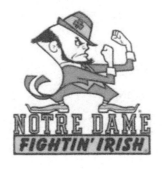

3rd Place Winner:   MICHIGAN STATE

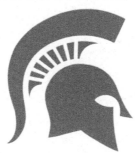

Runner Up:   YALE UNIVERSITY

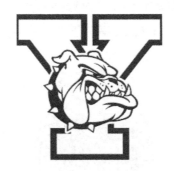

Other Great Schools:

UNIVERSITY OF COLORADO: BOULDER

KENT STATE UNIVERSITY

IOWA STATE UNIVERSITY

UNIVERSITY OF TENNESSEE

ITHACA COLLEGE

UNIVERSITY OF CONNECTICUT

UNIVERSITY OF ARIZONA

UNIVERSITY OF NEW HAMPSHIRE

GEORGETOWN UNIVERSITY

COLUMBIA UNIVERSITY

NC STATE UNIVERSITY

OREGON STATE UNIVERSITY

TOWSON UNIVERSITY

CLARK UNIVERSITY

CARLETON COLLEGE

# CELIAC SURVEY

We polled over 600 people with celiac disease
with the intent to make you feel not so alone.

## Have you gained or lost weight on a gluten free diet?

66%  Gained weight

34% Lost weight

Presented by The 2021 Gluten Free Buyers Guide

## YOU'RE NOT ALONE

# National Restaurant Chains

## 11th Annual Gluten Free Awards

1st Place Winner:   P.F. Changs

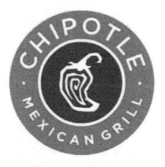

2nd Place Winner:   Chipotle

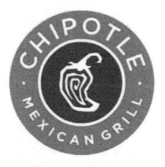

3rd Place Winner:   Chick-fil-A

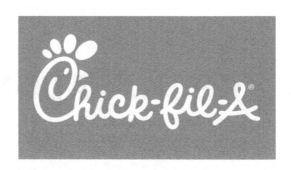

Runner Up:   Red Robin

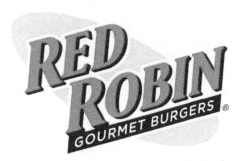

Other Great Restaurants:

Outback Steakhouse

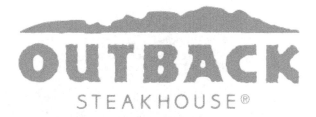

Jersey Mike's

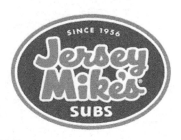

California Pizza Kitchen
The Bonefish Grill
True Food Kitchen

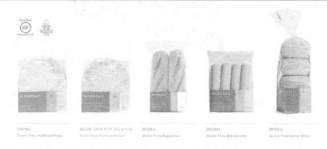

# MYBREAD
### GLUTEN FREE BAKERY

## Make MYBREAD Your Bread™

MYBREAD® is a 100% dedicated gluten-free, wholesale bakery located in Racine, WI. We differentiate ourselves by making all of our products are vegan and free from dairy, eggs, nuts and soy. All of our products are certified gluten-free by the Gluten Intolerance Group and Kosher by the Chicago Rabbinical Council.

ORIGINAL
Gluten Free Flatbread Pizza

ANCIENT GRAIN WITH CHIA & FLAX
Gluten Free Flatbread Pizza

ORIGINAL
Gluten Free Baguettes

ORIGINAL
Gluten Free Breadsticks

ORIGINAL
Gluten Free Dinner Rolls

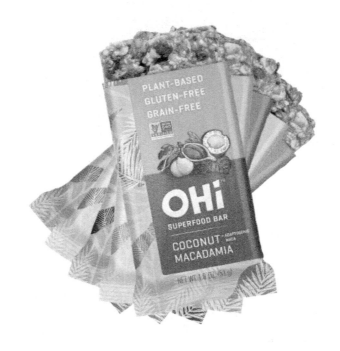

# Summer Camps

## 11th Annual Gluten Free Awards

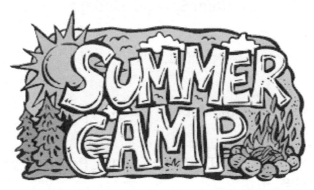

1st Place Winner: Gluten-Free Overnight Camp Middleville, Michigan

2nd Place Winner: The Great Gluten Escape at Gilmont Gilmer, Texas

3rd Place Winner:  GIG (Gluten Intolerance Group) Kids Camp East Camp Kanata Wake Forest, North Carolina

Runner Up:  Gluten Detectives Camp (Day Camp) Bloomington, Minnesota

Other Great Camps:

Camp Celiac Livermore, California

Timber Lake Camp Shandaken, New York

CDF Camp Gluten-Free™ Camp Fire Camp Nawakwa San Bernardino Mountains, CA

Camp Weekaneatit Warm Springs, Georgia

Camp Blue Spruce - Portland, OR

Gluten-Free Fun CampMaple Lake, Minnesota

International Sports Training Camp Pocono Mountains, Pennsylvania

Camp Celiac North Scituate, Rhode Island

Camp Celiac Strong - Hunt, NY

Foundation for Children & Youth with Diabetes Camp UTADA West Jordan, Utah

Camp Emerson Hinsdale, Massachusetts

Appel Farm Arts Camp Elmer, New Jersey

Clear Creek Camp Green' s Canyon, Utah (Serves Alpine School District children)

Emma Kaufmann Camp Morgantown, West Virginia

Camp Silly-Yak Brigadoon Village Aylesford, Nova Scotia

Camp Eagle Hill Elizaville, New York

Camp TAG Lebanon, Ohio at YMCA's Camp Kern

Camp TAG - Williamstown, New Jersey

GIG Kids Camp West Camp Sealth Vashon Island, Washington

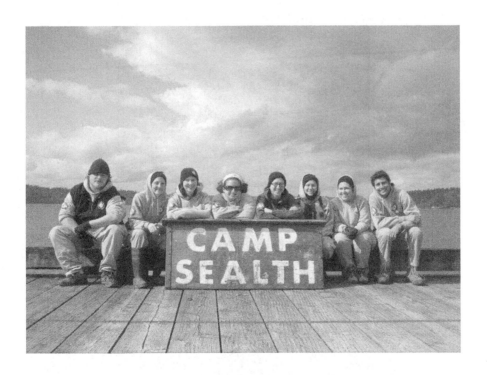

# Vacation Destinations

## 11ᵗʰ Annual Gluten Free Awards

1ˢᵗ Place Winner:   Walt Disney World, FL

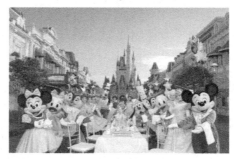

2ⁿᵈ Place Winner:   Italy

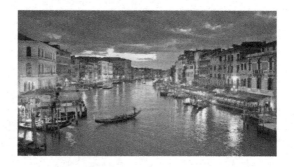

3ʳᵈ Place Winner:   New York City

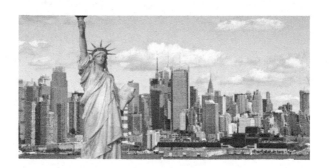

Runner Up:    Portland, OR

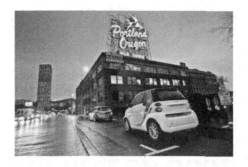

Other Great Destinations:

Royal Caribbean Cruises

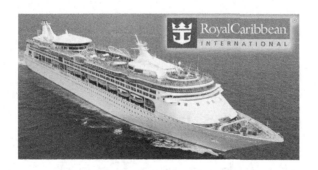

Disneyland, CA

London, England

Disney Cruises

Sandals

# CELIAC SURVEY

We polled over 600 people with celiac disease with the intent to make you feel not so alone.

## What food do you miss the most?

#1 Take Out Pizza

#2 Pastries

#3 Fried Chicken

#4 Chinese Food

Presented by The 2021 Gluten Free Buyers Guide

## YOU'RE NOT ALONE

# Magazine & Books

# Books

## 11ᵗʰ Annual Gluten Free Awards

1ˢᵗ Place Winner: The First Year: Celiac Disease and Living Gluten-Free: An Essential Guide for the Newly Diagnosed: Jules Shepard

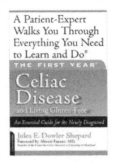

2ⁿᵈ Place Winner: Gluten Is My Bitch: Rants, Recipes, and Ridiculousness for the Gluten-Free by April Peveteaux

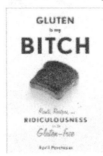

3ʳᵈ Place Winner: Celiac and the Beast: A Love Story Between a Gluten-Free Girl, Her Genes, and a Broken Digestive Tract by Erica Dermer

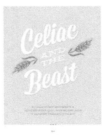

Runner Up: Gluten Freedom: The Nation's Leading Expert Offers the Essential Guide to a Healthy, Gluten-Free Lifestyle by Alessio Fasano (Author), Susie Flaherty (Contributor)

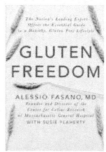

Other Great Books:

Undoctored: Why Health Care Has Failed You and How You Can Become Smarter Than Your Doctor by William Davis

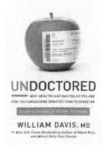

Dough Nation by Nadine Grzeskowiak

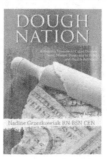

# NEW Gluten Free Heirloom Snack Crackers from PIPCORN!

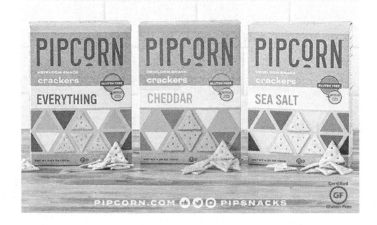

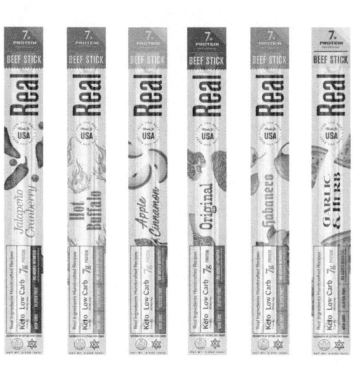

# Children's Books

## 11th Annual Gluten Free Awards

1st Place Winner:  Eat Like a Dinosaur: Recipe & Guidebook for Gluten-free Kids by Paleo Parents and Elana Amsterdam

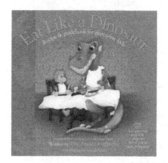

2nd Place Winner:  Everyone's Got Something: My First Year with Celiac Disease by Hallie Rose Katzman, Rayna Mae Katzman

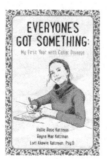

3rd Place Winner:  Dear Celiac by Kristen Adam

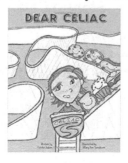

Runner Up:   The GF Kid: A Celiac Disease Survival Guide by Melissa London and Eric Glickman

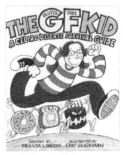

Other Great Books:

Wheat-Free, Gluten-Free Cookbook for Kids and Busy Adults by Connie Sarros

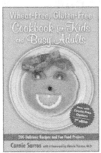

Eating Gluten-Free with Emily: A Story for Children with Celiac Disease by Bonnie J. Kruszka and Richard S. Cihlar

Aidan the Wonder Kid Who Could Not Be Stopped: A Food Allergy and Intolerance Story by Dan Carsten and Colleen Brunetti

Gordy and the Magic Diet by Kim Diersen (Author), April Runge (Author), Carrie Hartman (Illustrator)

The Gluten Glitch by Stasie John and Kevin Cannon

# Cookbooks

## 11th Annual Gluten Free Awards

1st Place Winner: Nearly Normal Cooking For Gluten-Free Eating: A Fresh Approach to Cooking and Living Without Wheat or Gluten by Jules E. D. Shepard and Alessio Fasano

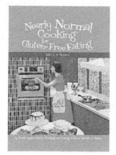

2nd Place Winner:  Gluten-Free on a Shoestring: 125 Easy Recipes for Eating Well on the Cheap by Nicole Hunn

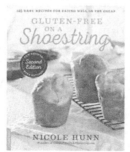

3rd Place Winner:  How Can It Be Gluten Free Cookbook Collection: 350+ Groundbreaking Recipes for All Your Favorites by America's Test Kitchen

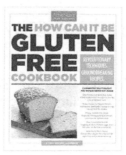

Runner Up: The Everything Gluten-Free & Dairy-Free Cookbook: 300 simple and satisfying recipes without gluten or dairy by Audrey Roberts

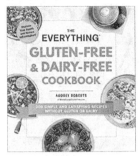

Other Great Cookbooks:

The Big Book of Gluten Free Baking by Paola Anna Miget

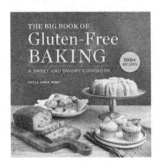

Wandering Palate, By Erika Schlick

101 Incredible Gluten-Free Recipes by Jennifer Bigler

The Autoimmune Paleo Cookbook: An Allergen-Free Approach to Managing Chronic Illness by Mickey Trescott

The Gluten-Free Kitchen: Over 135 Delicious Recipes for People with Gluten Intolerance or Wheat Allergy by Roben Ryberg

The Warm Kitchen by Amy Fothergill

No Gluten, No Problem Pizza: 75+ Recipes for Every Craving—from Thin Crust to Deep Dish, New York to Naples

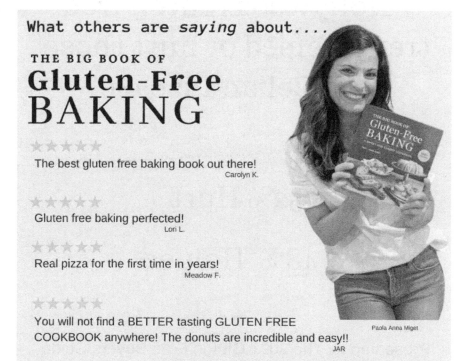

# Celiac Survey

We polled over 600 people with celiac disease with the intent to make you feel not so alone.

Do you think the celebrity / Hollywood gluten free trend helped or hurt those with Celiac Disease?

52% Hurt

48% Helped

Presented by The 2021 Gluten Free Buyers Guide

## YOU'RE NOT ALONE

# Magazines

## 11th Annual Gluten Free Awards

1st Place Winner:   Simply Gluten Free

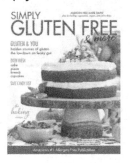

2nd Place Winner:   GFF Magazine

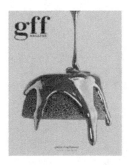

3rd Place Winner:   Allergic Living

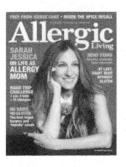

Runner Up:   Paleo Magazine

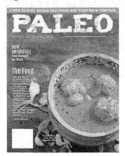

Other Great Magazines:

yum.

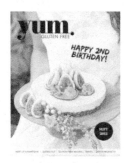

Gluten Free Heaven – UK

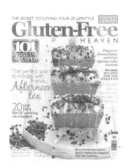

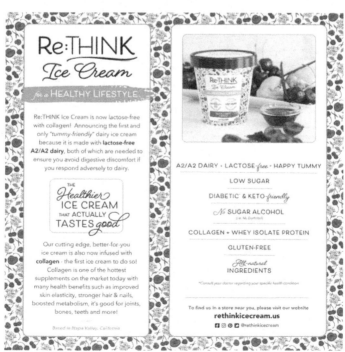

# Media

# Blogs & Websites

## 11th Annual Gluten Free Awards

1st Place Winner:   Mama Knows Gluten Free

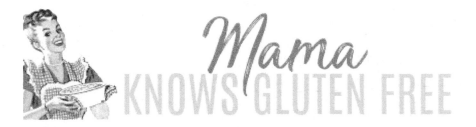

2nd Place Winner:   MealHacks.com

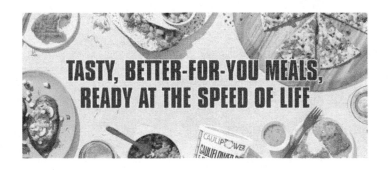

3rd Place Winner:   Gluten Free Follow Me

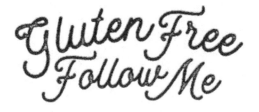

Runner Up:    Gluten Free Watch Dog

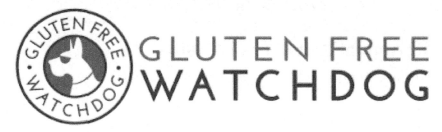

Other Great Blogs & Websites:

Livingfreelyglutenfree.com

Healthy GF Family

What The Fork Food Blog

Nom Nom Paleo

Celiac Project

The Paleo Mom

Stayglutenfree.com

Gluten Free Globetrotter

The Gluten Free Travelers

Cure Celiac Disease.org

Gluten Free RN

# Expos

## 11<sup>th</sup> Annual Gluten Free Awards

1<sup>st</sup> Place Winner: The Nourished Festival (formerly GFAF Expo)

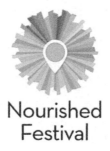

2<sup>nd</sup> Place Winner: Natural Expo West

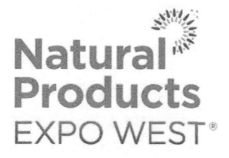

3<sup>rd</sup> Place Winner: CDF National Education & Gluten-Free Expo

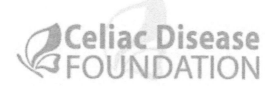

Runner Up:   Natural Expo East

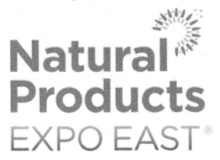

Other Great Expos:

Fancy Food Summer Show
Fancy Food Winter Show

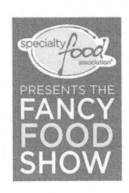

# CELIAC SURVEY

We polled over 600 people with celiac disease with the intent to make you feel not so alone.

## Have people made fun of the gluten free diet in front of you?

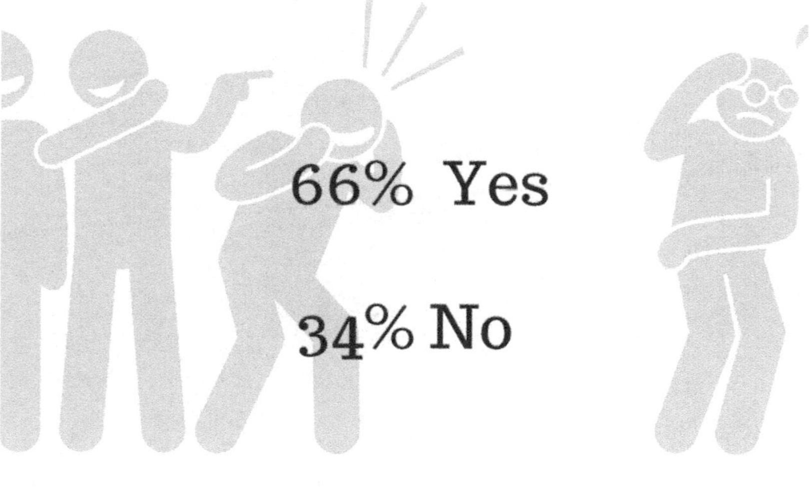

66% Yes

34% No

Presented by The 2021 Gluten Free Buyers Guide

# YOU'RE NOT ALONE

# Mobile Apps

## 11th Annual Gluten Free Awards

1st Place Winner:   Find Me Gluten Free

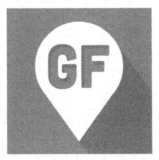

2nd Place Winner:   The Gluten Free Scanner

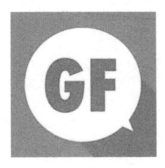

3rd Place Winner:   Spokin

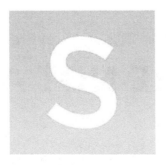

Runner Up:   Dedicated Gluten Free

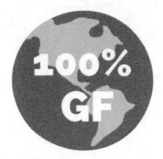

Other Great Apps:

GF Plate

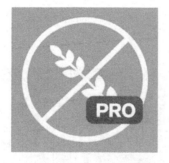

Now Find Gluten Free

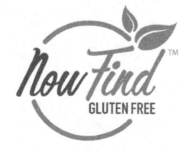

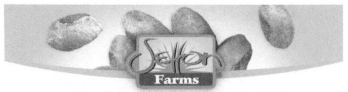
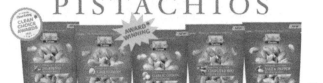

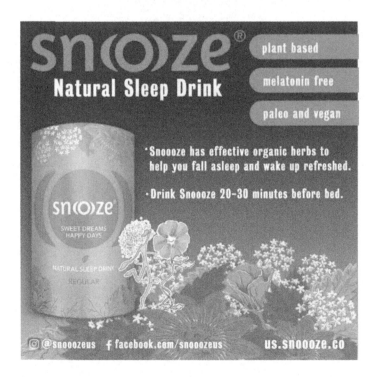

# Nonprofits

## 11<sup>th</sup> Annual Gluten Free Awards

1<sup>st</sup> Place Winner:   Celiac Disease Foundation (CDF)

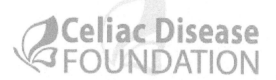

2<sup>nd</sup> Place Winner:   Gluten Intolerance Group of North America (GIG)

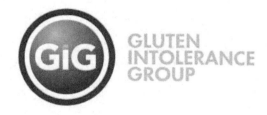

3<sup>rd</sup> Place Winner:   Beyond Celiac

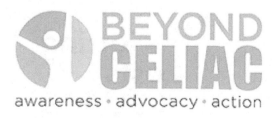

Runner Up:   National Celiac Disease Society (NCDS)

N A T I O N A L
C E L I A C
D I S E A S E
S O C I E T Y

Other Great Nonprofits:

Celiac Support Association (CSA) (formerly Celiac Sprue Association)

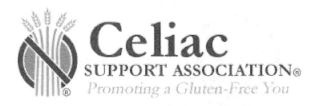

Cutting Costs for Celiacs Food Equality Initiative

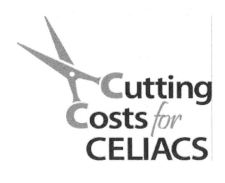

# Online Resources

## 11th Annual Gluten Free Awards

1st Place Winner:   Celiac.org

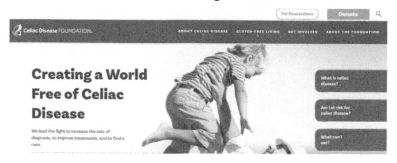

2nd Place Winner:   GlutenFreeWatchDog.org

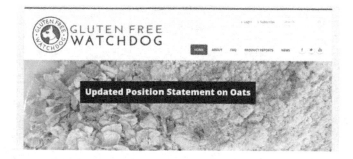

3rd Place Winner:   Beyondceliac.org

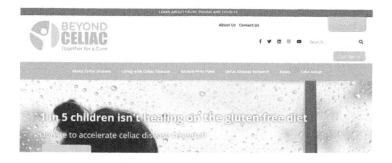

Runner Up:    Glutenfreefollowme.com

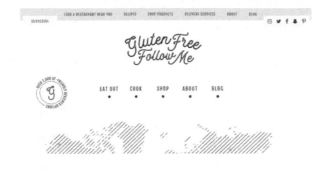

Other Great Resources:

Gluten.org

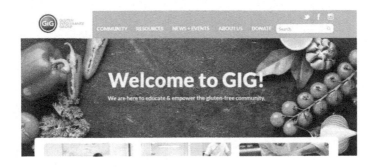

Everybody Eats! - Naomi Poe YouTube Cooking Tutorials

CeliacCentral.org

Cureceliacdisease.org

# CELIAC SURVEY

We polled over 600 people with celiac disease with the intent to make you feel not so alone.

## Would you recommend Celiac Disease screening (blood test) for all?

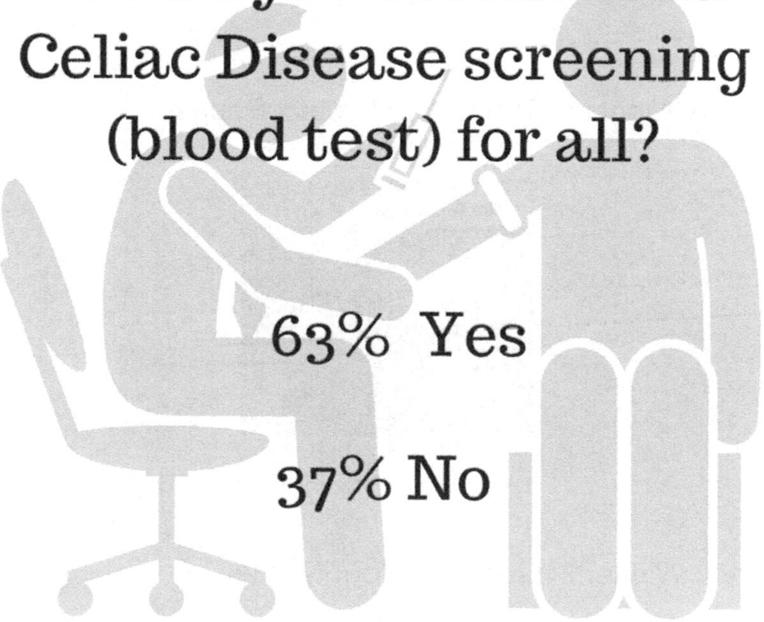

63% Yes

37% No

Presented by The 2021 Gluten Free Buyers Guide

## YOU'RE NOT ALONE

# Podcasts

## 11<sup>th</sup> Annual Gluten Free Awards

1<sup>st</sup> Place Winner:   The Gluten Free News

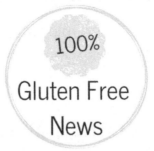

2<sup>nd</sup> Place Winner:   The Celiac Project Podcast

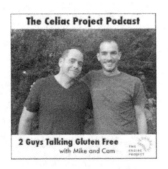

3<sup>rd</sup> Place Winner:   Listen To Your Mother

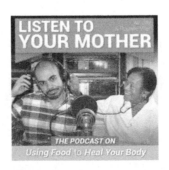

Runner Up:   Gluten Free RN

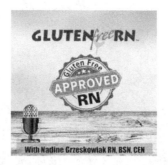

Other Great Podcasts:

Serving Celiacs

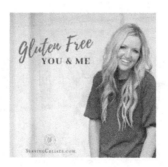

# Online Stores

## 11ᵗʰ Annual Gluten Free Awards

1st Place Winner:   Amazon

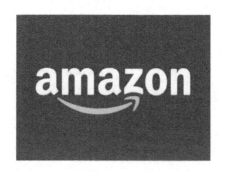

2nd Place Winner:   Thrive Market

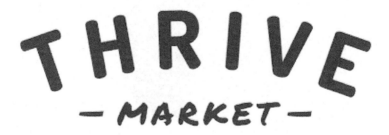

3rd Place Winner:   Gluten Free Mall

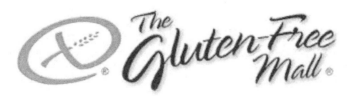

Runner Up:   Vitacost

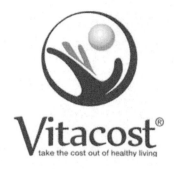

Other Great Stores:

Walmart Online

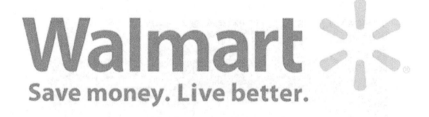

Target Online

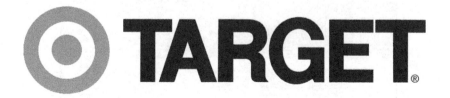

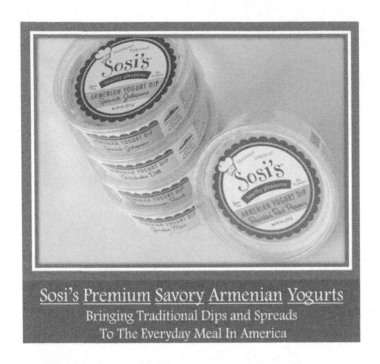

## Sosi's Premium Savory Armenian Yogurts
### Bringing Traditional Dips and Spreads
### To The Everyday Meal In America

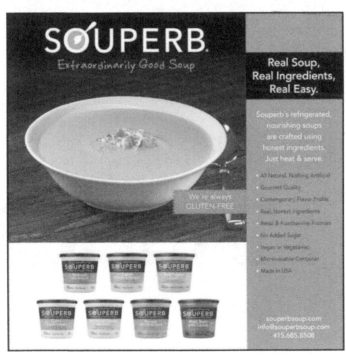

# Social Media Platforms

## 11th Annual Gluten Free Awards

1st Place Winner:   Facebook

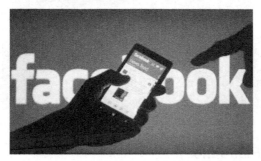

2nd Place Winner:   Instagram

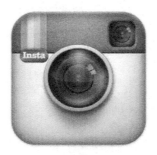

3rd Place Winner:   Pinterest

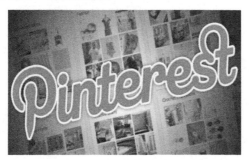

Runner Up:   Twitter

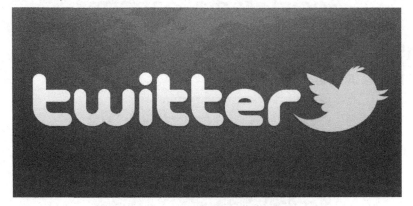

Other Great Platforms:

Tik Tok

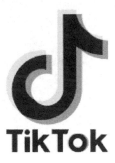

Freedible

Meet-Up

Linked In

# CELIAC SURVEY

We polled over 600 people with celiac disease with the intent to make you feel not so alone.

## Is it harder to date others when you are on a gluten free diet?

63% Yes

37% No

Presented by The 2021 Gluten Free Buyers Guide

## YOU'RE NOT ALONE

# Other

# Comfort Foods

## 11<sup>th</sup> Annual Gluten Free Awards

1<sup>st</sup> Place Winner:   CAULIPOWER Three Cheese Cauliflower Crust Pizza

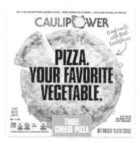

2<sup>nd</sup> Place Winner:   Trader Joe's Gluten Free Mac & Cheese (Frozen)

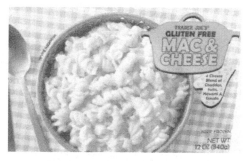

3<sup>rd</sup> Place Winner:   Justin's Organic White Chocolate Peanut Butter Cup

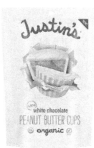

Runner Up: Jolly Llama Dairy-Free Gluten-Free Premium Vanilla Sandwich

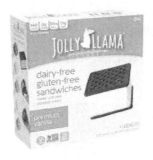

Other Great Products:

Mr. Lee's Hong Kong Street-Style Beef Rice Noodle Soup

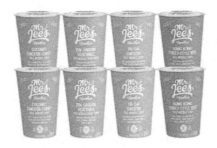

EPIC Sea Salt & Pepper Pork Rinds

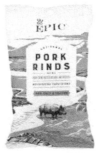

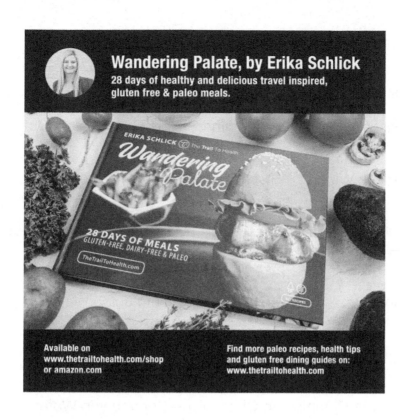
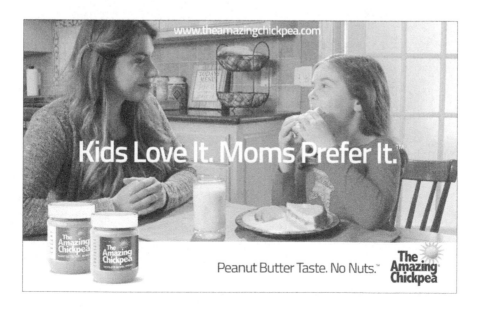

# Communion Products

## 11th Annual Gluten Free Awards

1st Place Winner:  Benedictine Sisters Communion Wafers


2nd Place Winner:  Gluten Free Hosts (glutenfreehosts.com)


3rd Place Winner:  The Gluten & Grain Free Gourmet Allergy Free Communion Wafers


Runner Up:  Ener G Gluten Free Communion Wafers


Other Great Products:


Celebrate Communion Gluten Free Communion Wafers

# New Products

## 11th Annual Gluten Free Awards

1st Place Winner:   CAULIPOWER Baja Style Riced Cauliflower

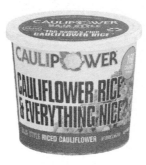

2nd Place Winner:   MYBREAD Soft Breadsticks

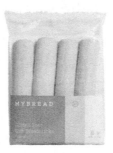

3rd Place Winner:   Mikey's Buffalo Chicken Pockets

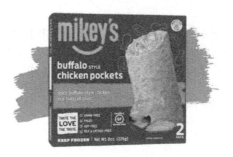

Runner Up: Jolly Llama Dairy-Free Gluten-Free Premium Vanilla Fudge Sundae Cone

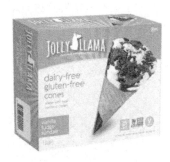

Other Great Products:

Mr. Lee's Hong Kong Street-Style Beef Rice Noodle Soup

Veggies Made Great Sausage, Egg & Cheese Frittata made with Beyond Meat®

GOODTO GO™ Double Chocolate Soft Baked Bar

ALDI-exclusive Park Street Deli Original Guacamole Mini Cups

ALDI-exclusive Park Street Deli Homestyle Guacamole Mini Cups

Bakery on Main Grain Free Clusters with MCT Oil

Gluten Free Complete™

Veggies Made Great Sausage & Pepper Frittata made with Beyond Meat®

ALDI-exclusive Park Street Deli Spicy Guacamole Mini Cups

GOODTO GO™ Vanilla Almond Soft Baked Bar

Wonder Drink Prebiotic Kombucha - Prickly Pear Cascara for Focus

Purecane™ Baking Sweetener

Real Jalapeño Cranberry Beef Stick

# CELIAC SURVEY

We polled over 600 people with celiac disease
with the intent to make you feel not so alone.

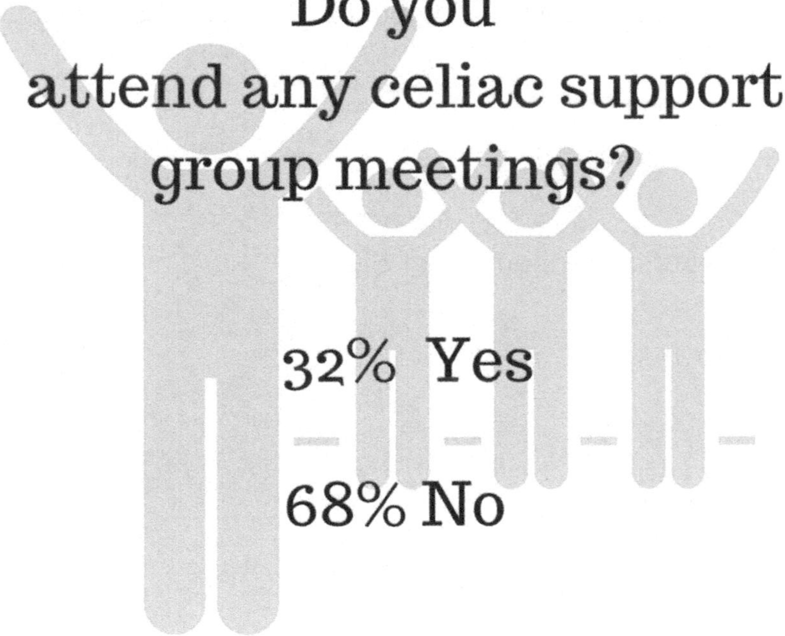

## Do you attend any celiac support group meetings?

32%  Yes

68% No

Presented by The 2021 Gluten Free Buyers Guide

## YOU'RE NOT ALONE

# Pasta, Sides, Soup & Sauces

# Macaroni and Cheese

## 11th Annual Gluten Free Awards

1st Place Winner:    Amy's Gluten Free Frozen Mac & Cheese

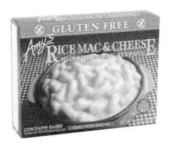

2nd Place Winner:    Trader Joe's Gluten Free Mac & Cheese

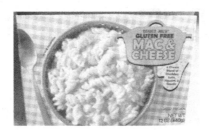

3rd Place Winner:    ALDI-exclusive liveGfree Gluten Free Shells & Cheese

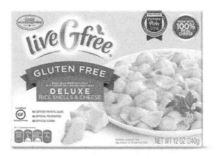

Runner Up:   Walmart -  Great Value Gluten-Free Macaroni & Cheese

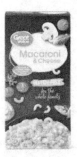

Other Great Products:

Banza Chickpea Pasta - High Protein Gluten Free Mac & Cheese

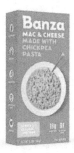

Lidl Gluten Free Rice Pasta & Cheddar Cheese

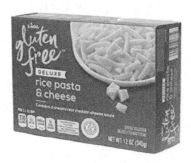

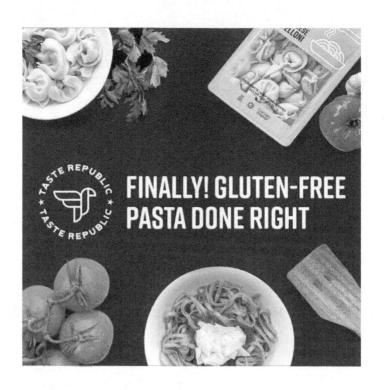

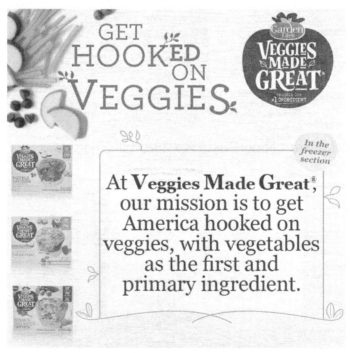

# Pastas

## 11th Annual Gluten Free Awards

1st Place Winner: Jovial Gluten Free Brown Rice Pasta Spaghetti

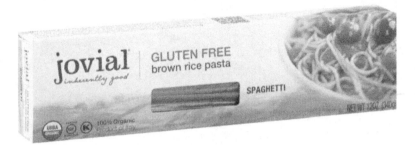

2nd Place Winner: Tinkyada Penne

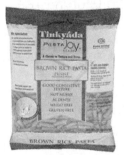

3rd Place Winner: Le Veneziane Fettucce

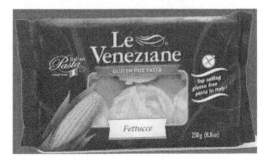

Runner Up:   ALDI-exclusive liveGfree Gluten Free Fettuccine

Other Great Products:

ALDI-exclusive liveGfree Gluten Free Linguine

Lidl Gluten Free Penne Pasta

Lidl Gluten Free Fusilli Pasta

Farabella BIO Rigatoni

# Sauces

## 11th Annual Gluten Free Awards

1st Place Winner:   San-J Organic Tamari Soy Sauce

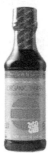

2nd Place Winner:   Rao's Homemade Marinara Sauce

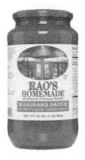

3rd Place Winner:   ALDI-exclusive Fusia Asian Stir Fry Sweet & Sour Sauce

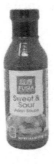

Runner Up:   Fody Original Barbecue Sauce

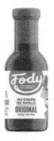

Other Great Products:

Fody Taco Sauce

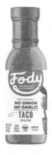

ALDI-exclusive Fusia Asian Style Bang Bang Restaurant Sauce

Fody Teriyaki Sauce & Marinade

ALDI-exclusive Cook House Indian Tikka Masala Sauce

# CELIAC SURVEY

We polled over 600 people with celiac disease with the intent to make you feel not so alone.

## Do you feel alone living the gluten free lifestyle?

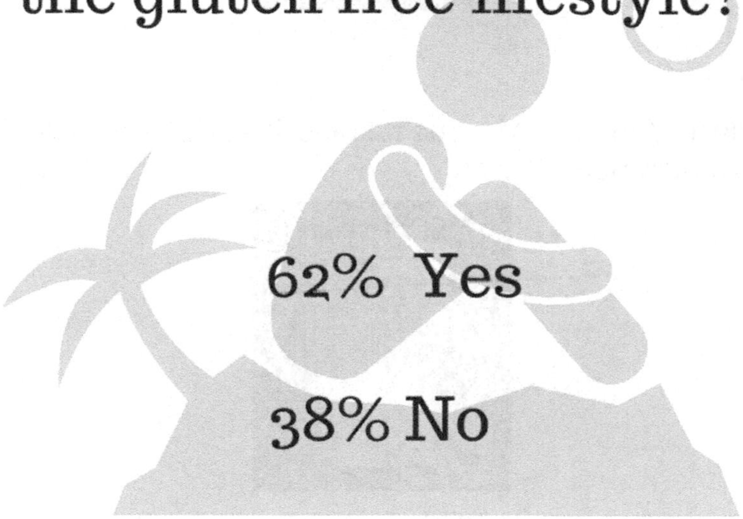

62% Yes

38% No

Presented by The 2021 Gluten Free Buyers Guide

## YOU'RE NOT ALONE

# Soup

## 11th Annual Gluten Free Awards

1st Place Winner: ALDI-exclusive Specially Selected Slow Cooked Baked Potato Soup with Applewood Smoked Uncured Bacon

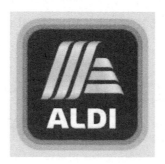

2nd Place Winner: Mr. Lee's Hong Kong Street-Style Beef Rice Noodle Soup

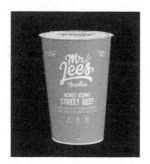

3rd Place Winner: ALDI-exclusive Specially Selected Slow Cooked Creamy Broccoli Cheddar Bisque

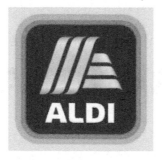

Runner Up: Golden Ladle Organic Gluten-Free Chicken Sipping Bone Broth

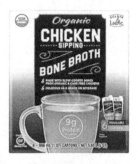

Other Great Products:

ALDI-exclusive Simply Nature Organic Lentil Soup

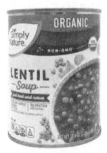

Parks and Nash Bone Broth Soup

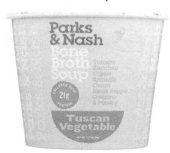

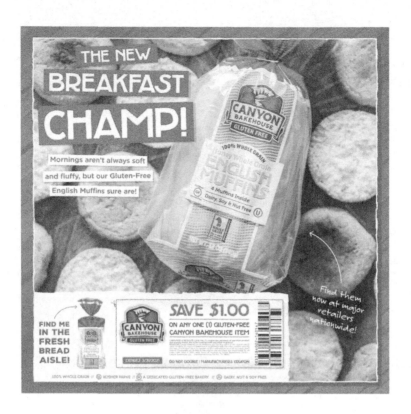

## Farabella BIO (Organic) Gluten Free Pasta

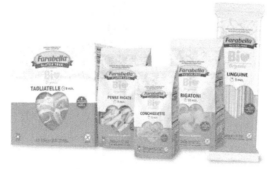

Tagliatelle - Penne Rigate - Conchigliette (small shells) - Rigatoni - Linguine

www. quattrobimbi.com - info@quattrobimbi.com - (866) 618-7759

# Stuffing

## 11th Annual Gluten Free Awards

1st Place Winner:   Trader Joe's Gluten Free Stuffing

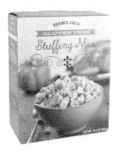

2nd Place Winner:   ALDI-exclusive liveGfree Gluten Free Chicken Stuffing

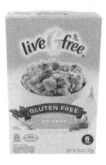

3rd Place Winner:   Aleia's Gluten Free Savory Stuffing Mix

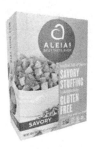

Runner Up:   Williams Sonoma Gluten-Free Stuffing

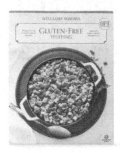

Other Great Products:

Aleia's Gluten Free Plain Stuffing Mix

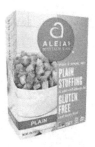

Gillian's Gluten Free Home Style Stuffing

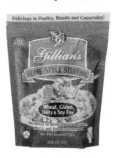

# Personalities

# Coral Barajas

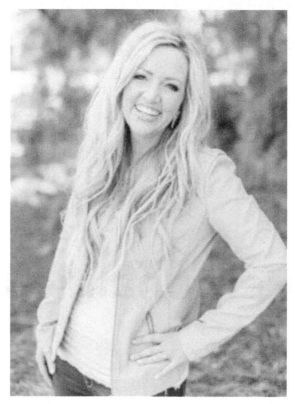

How long have you been gluten free?

6 years

Do you have any other dietary restrictions?

Dairy sensitivity

What has been your biggest challenge thus far?

Eating out safely

Where is your favorite place to eat?

In n out

Do you have any gluten related pet peeves?

When extended family won't get tested when clearly they are sick.

How has the Covid quarantine changed your diet habits?

It has been a great change as we don't have many gatherings- less chances for my kids and I to be sick

Do you have a gluten horror story?

All the painful nights of watching my kids be sick after being glutened!

What has been the biggest change since you became gluten free?

Awareness for what I am eating!

In ten years, a gluten free diet will be···

Understood and more convenient!

What is the best advice you received?

It gets easier with time to navigate

What is the best way for people to connect with you?

@servingceliacs on IG

# Christina P. Kantzavelos

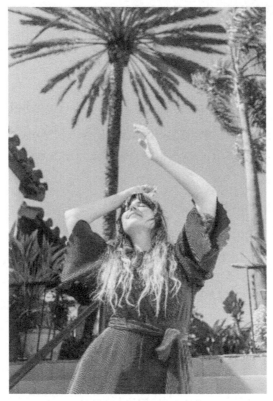

How long have you been gluten free?

Since 2012.


Do you have any other dietary restrictions?

Dairy, and mostly soy, refined sugar, and alcohol. None of which restricts how delicious the food I eat is!


What has been your biggest challenge thus far?

Preparation. I've learned time, and time again, that if you do not adequately prepare for trips, social events, surprises (like traffic), non-GF restaurants, that you may end up in challenging situations, including feeling hangry or hypoglycemic. This requires conducting adequate research and having plenty of snacks on hand at all times... In your bag, in your car, everywhere. I'm much better than I used to be, but I still have my moments.

Where is your favorite place to eat?

My kitchen, always. I can be endlessly creative, use organic, quality, and nutrient-dense ingredients, and do it on my own time. However, San Diego has some pretty awesome 100% gluten-free spots that I enjoy frequenting, such as Nectarine Grove and Healthy Creations. Follow @glutenfree_sandiego_meetups for the best-of spots in San Diego, CA!

Do you have any gluten related pet peeves?

I have two. One is that many restaurants/places do not seem to take my gluten-free/celiac requests seriously unless I call it a "gluten allergy." The second pet-peeve is when restaurants claim their menu items are gluten-free when they are cooked in the same oil/area without switching anything out first. I try to breathe through both and make them teachable moments, however, they are still quite frustrating.

How has the Covid quarantine changed your diet habits?

I mostly ate at home prior to Covid-19, so it's actually no different. I safely shop at my local health food/grocery stores, and the farmer's market. And I once in a while get food-to-go from my favorite spots. I do look forward to freely breaking (gluten-free) bread with friends and family again.

Do you have a gluten horror story?

I thankfully haven't had one of those for myself in a while. Though, my mom was diagnosed last year, and watching her make not-so-great decisions, and paying the price for them afterward is pretty horrific to watch.

What has been the biggest change since you became gluten free?

Feeling sharper, and all-around better. I'm grateful that I found out as early as I did, and had/have the resources to support my diet and lifestyle.

In ten years, a gluten free diet will be···

Normalized, and better understood. It will be both faster and easier to get a diagnosis. There will be more options, public awareness, and it will be safer and take less effort (dare I say less preparation?) to go about a normal routine and do anything you choose. There will also be more research studies, and there may even be treatment options for celiac disease.

What is the best advice you received?

"Nothing tastes better than feeling good." They were 100% right.

What is the best way for people to connect with you?

www.buenqamino.com

www.instagram.com/buenqamino

www.facebook.com/buenqamio

www.twitter.com/buenqamino

www.pinterest.com/buenqamino

hello@buenqamino.com

# Jackie McEwan

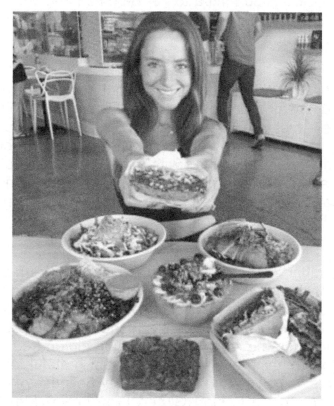

How long have you been gluten free?

8+ years

Do you have any other dietary restrictions?

Just gluten

What has been your biggest challenge thus far?

My biggest challenge was when I found out that I had to follow a gluten-free diet. I was completely overwhelmed. I did not even know what gluten was! I had to figure out what foods I could eat, what foods I had to avoid, and the nuances in between. I wished I had a go-to guide to tell me all I needed to know about following a gluten-free diet. This manual did not yet exist, so I did a ton of research and learned how to maneuver being gluten-free at restaurants and in my own kitchen.

In March 2014, I started to post about some of the gluten-free foods I was eating on Instagram. Surprisingly to me, my posts were met with great reception. People I had never met were asking me for more tips on gluten-free friendly eateries, products, and recipes, and I was more than happy to continue to make these discoveries. I was getting so many questions that I knew I needed to put all this information in one place rather than just Instagram.

In September 2014, I taught myself how to make a website, and I launched glutenfreefollowme.com! I wish I had something like Gluten Free Follow Me to guide me through my new gluten-free diet eight years ago, but I am glad I can be a guide for others now! At the time, going gluten-free seemed like the worst thing ever. However, I am grateful for it now. Knowledge is power, and I am healthier because of it. Going gluten-free led me to start Gluten Free Follow Me. If I had not become gluten-free, I would probably still be working in finance in New York City. My quest to find gluten-free foods developed into a full-time passion, and I could not be happier with how it all turned out!

Where is your favorite place to eat?

I have many favorites! A few of my faves are: Posh Pop Bakeshop in NYC, Vibe Organic Kitchen in Newport Beach, and Petunia's Pies & Pastries in Portland. Many more on glutenfreefollowme.com/restaurants :)

Do you have any gluten related pet peeves?

When someone says that they could never give up gluten. When you have to, yes you can! And honestly, it's not that hard, especially nowadays. There are so many amazing options.

How has the Covid quarantine changed your diet habits?

I can't say that it has! I still eat fairly balanced with lots of fruits and veggies, and my fair share of chocolate, baked goods, and sweets :)

Do you have a gluten horror story?

Back when I was working in NYC, I went out to lunch at a restaurant that is now closed. I told the hostess, manager, and waitress that I was gluten-free. They went through the menu with me and told me which options were safe for me to eat. I ended up ordering the nachos as an appetizer. I had just taken my first bite of the nachos when the manager ran over to tell me that the nachos were not actually gluten-free. The chips had cross contamination in the fryer. I couldn't believe it! It was even more frustrating because I had asked the right questions. Thankfully, something like this hasn't happened to me again.

What has been the biggest change since you became gluten free?

Every year, it becomes easier to follow a gluten-free diet! It's more straightforward to find gluten-free foods. Supermarkets and stores now have gluten-free sections, and food labeling has gotten better. Products market themselves to the gluten-free consumer. Some brands have even modified their ingredients in order to make their products gluten-free. The restaurant scene has become more sensitive to people who follow a gluten-free diet. Some restaurants have menus that indicate which items are gluten-free, and this definitely wasn't the case seven years ago. Waiters are usually well-versed in how to accommodate dietary needs, unlike a few years ago when the majority of waiters didn't even know what gluten was.

In ten years, a gluten free diet will be⋯

Even more widespread. I see the gluten-free world continuing down the path of increased awareness. I've eaten at 75 completely gluten-free eateries, and I expect to see even more 100% gluten-free eateries in the future. I predict that the number of people who go gluten-free will keep on multiplying. After all, gluten-free food truly tastes good now, and it's a healthier way to live.

What is the best advice you received?

Make something people want.

What is the best way for people to connect with you?

Instagram: @glutenfree.followme

Twitter: @glutenfreefm

Facebook: Gluten Free Follow Me

Blog: glutenfreefollowme.com

# Jennifer Fitzpatrick

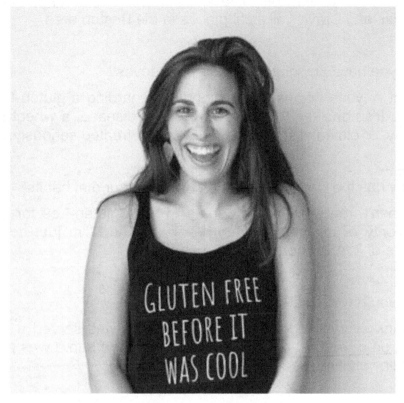

How long have you been gluten free?

11 years - since my diagnosis with celiac disease.


Do you have any other dietary restrictions?

No - just a slight lactose-intolerance.


What has been your biggest challenge thus far?

My biggest challenge with eating gluten-free was healing my gut in the beginning. Celiac disease led to many other complications like SIBO, IBS, and candida overgrowth.

Where is your favorite place to eat?

I prefer to eat at home! I love to cook and bake gluten-free. But if I'm heading out, I love Twist Cafe & Bakery, Papa Razzi, and Crave - all local places in the Boston area.


Do you have any gluten related pet peeves?

Yes! Anyone who is condescending regarding a gluten-free diet. It's not a fad for those with celiac disease, a wheat allergy, or gluten allergy. It deserves to be treated seriously.


How has the Covid quarantine changed your diet habits?

It hasn't, really! I already cook and bake gluten-free for the majority of my meals every week, but now I'm just doing more of it. And I don't mind!


Do you have a gluten horror story?

I think everyone does! Mine was when I was served a hot dog on a regular bun instead of a gluten-free bun. I was projectile vomiting for 3 hours. It was awful.


What has been the biggest change since you became gluten free?

My confidence and resilience. I'm now empowered to eat safely both at home and around the world because I make a point to be prepared and advocate for myself. It's how I spent 6 months backpacking abroad last year safely and successfully!


In ten years, a gluten free diet will be···

Since I've seen the improvement of the gluten-free diet from my diagnosis until now, which was over a decade ago, I'm sure the diet will have more options, products, and protocols. I think it continues to improve every year - slowly, but surely.

What is the best advice you received?

Not being able to eat gluten doesn't mean your life is over. Adapt, learn, and seek support!

What is the best way for people to connect with you?

I'm on Instagram @jefinner589 and my website, www.thenomadicfitzpatricks.com has gluten-free recipes, products & guides to eat and explore with celiac disease. Hope to see you there!

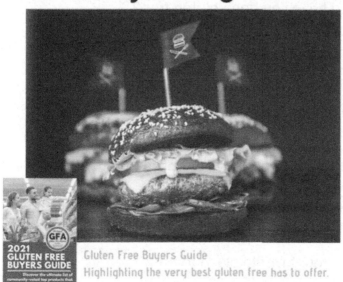

## You know you are gluten free

2021 GLUTEN FREE BUYERS GUIDE

Gluten Free Buyers Guide
Highlighting the very best gluten free has to offer.

## When your bun costs more than the burger

# Jennifer Bigler

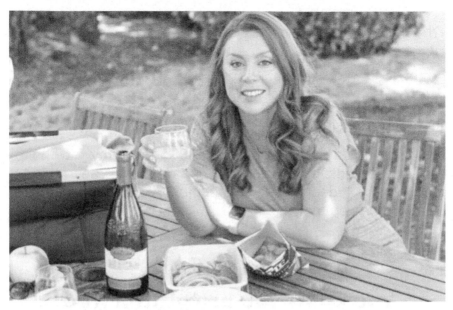

How long have you been gluten free?

9 years

Do you have any other dietary restrictions?

Yes, lactose free

What has been your biggest challenge thus far?

Eating out or traveling and managing all of my families food intolerances- gluten, dairy, corn, and some nuts.

Where is your favorite place to eat?

It depends where I am, but New Cascadia pizza in Portland is the best.

Do you have any gluten related pet peeves?

Mostly when people make fun of it, or do not take it seriously.

How has the Covid quarantine changed your diet habits?

At first we weren't able to get a lot of ingredients we wanted, so we had to meal plan based on what was available. Now everything is mostly back to normal.

Do you have a gluten horror story?

When we were at one of our favorite gf bakeries we grabbed some ice cream sandwiches for purchase and we only read the ingredients because my son can't have corn. They contained regular flour and they had to pull them all out of the freezer. I hope no one ate them and got sick.

What has been the biggest change since you became gluten free?

How many options are available at the store and I don't have to explain what gluten is anymore. 9 years ago no one knew what is was.

In ten years, a gluten free diet will be···

Hopefully not a fad anymore and taken very seriously. Everyone will be more educated and there will be options at most places.

What is the best advice you received?

Listen to your body.

What is the best way for people to connect with you?

Instagram @livingfreelyglutenfree

# Jules Shepard

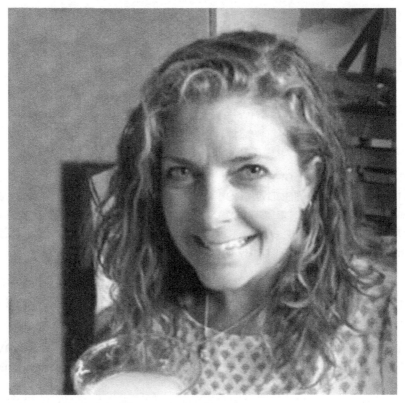

How long have you been gluten free?

21 years!


Do you have any other dietary restrictions?

No dairy, mostly vegan and I don't do any meat.


What has been your biggest challenge thus far?

Personally, my challenge has just been if I want to eat out. I can really make anything I want for myself and my family at home, so for travel or socializing with friends at a restaurant, it can be a bit challenging, awkward and sometimes very stressful to put my trust in a restaurant instead.

Where is your favorite place to eat?

Haha ... speaking of trusting someone else! My favorite place to eat besides home (!) is no longer open. It was one of the places I looked forward to visiting when I traveled out west for gluten-free shows or to see friends, and I learned that due to the pandemic, it closed its doors. I was so sad to learn of its demise, as well as that of so many other dedicated gluten free restaurants around the country. I truly hope that we'll see a return of dedicated GF restaurants again one day once the country recovers.

Do you have any gluten related pet peeves?

Doesn't everyone?!

It still annoys me when people think that gluten is a fad or that being gluten free is some kind of choice for us. It also annoys me that there are so many food companies out there who still make bad gluten free food! It's like they don't eat their own products!! Cheap ingredients made bad food -- it's a pretty simple concept. But the end result is that gluten free food still has a bad name because of it. Gluten free food can be super delicious and people need to know that, but they have to be exposed to the right ingredients and products, so there's still a lot of work to be done.

How has the Covid quarantine changed your diet habits?

It hasn't changed my habits much, since we hardly ever ate out before. But we actually have tried to order take out MORE than we did before just to help restaurants stay in business. So I guess in that way it has changed our habits a bit, but there aren't a lot of gluten free restaurant options near us, so I suppose the ones nearby are getting more used to seeing our name pop up on their caller ID!

Do you have a gluten horror story?

How many do you want? I already told you I've been gluten free for 21 years, so that's a lot of time for horror stories! I have plenty to have accumulated during that time, but also before I was diagnosed and during the 10 years I was still eating gluten before I was diagnosed and was so sick. Gluten and I really don't get along very well at all! Pretty much anyone reading this can think on their own horror stories and I've been right there with you. If you want some more specifics, I outline several in my book, The First Year: Celiac Disease and Living Gluten Free.

What has been the biggest change since you became gluten free?

People in the general population actually have heard of gluten and celiac disease! When I was diagnosed, no one (including myself) had even heard of gluten. So there have been many, many changes. There are products on the market that are made FOR people eating gluten free, products are labeled and certified gluten free, there are gluten free menus, there are blood tests for celiac disease, there is a genetic test for celiac disease ... so many changes!

In ten years, a gluten free diet will be⋯

Completely mainstream.

What is the best advice you received?

I didn't. There was no one to give me advice when I was told I had to go gluten free. Literally, my doctor told me I had celiac disease and couldn't eat gluten, and then he said he thought it was in bread, but wasn't sure what it was. There were no nutritionists at the time to help me, no internet resources, no books to speak of ... it was a real wasteland of information. I ate Rice Krispies cereal until I figured out for myself that malt flavoring contained barley which also contained gluten. Then I ate Peppermint Patties because I thought they didn't have any gluten in them. And rice. I ate lots of rice. It was a dark time for me! (Don't worry, I finally figured it out!)

What is the best way for people to connect with you?

@gfJules on FB, IG & Pinterest and @THEgfJules on Twitter or through my blog gfJules.com.

## You know you are gluten free

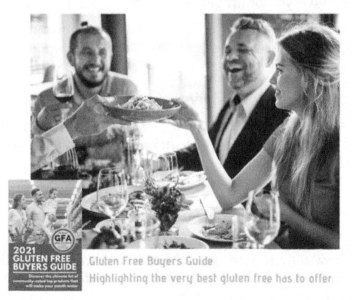

Gluten Free Buyers Guide
Highlighting the very best gluten free has to offer.

## When you eat before you go out to eat

# Erica Dermer

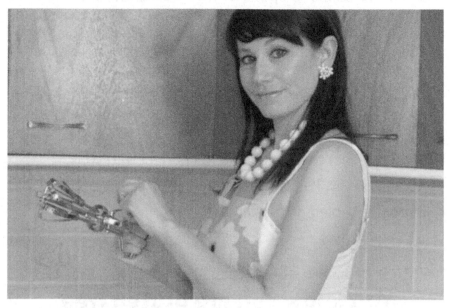

How long have you been gluten free?

10-ish years! There were a few years of on and off diagnoses while I was waiting on a celiac disease true diagnosis!

Do you have any other dietary restrictions?

I can't eat beef - haven't had it in 12 or so years. I've cut out dairy for about 5-6 years, and eggs on and off for years. I now eat baked eggs (like eggs in bread).

What has been your biggest challenge thus far?

Fighting the misinformation of the internet! Unfortunately, too many still view gluten free as a "diet to try" when in reality it's a medical diet that should be given by a medical professional after a celiac disease screening.

Where is your favorite place to eat?

We're so lucky to have so many great dedicated gluten-free restaurants and bakeries here in Phoenix, and gluten-free friendly restaurants. I don't have a favorite - I just love to eat!

Do you have any gluten related pet peeves?

Brands that don't have easily accessible information on their website or social media about how their product is made and how/where they source their ingredients.

How has the Covid quarantine changed your diet habits?

I have been buying a lot more products online and in bulk! However, you have to be really careful to not try new products in bulk - or else you have a LOT of something you don't like!

Do you have a gluten horror story?

Most of the "horror stories" revolve around front of the house servers or managers that don't understand the seriousness of making a restaurant item safe for those with celiac, after claiming it is "gluten free."

What has been the biggest change since you became gluten free?

We are so lucky - in 2020 we have so many great gluten-free products out there. Seriously, name a product and we have a gluten-free replacement out there. We've grown so much!

In ten years, a gluten free diet will be···

Hopefully better understood as a medically-necessary diet.

What is the best advice you received?

It will get easier, it just takes time.

What is the best way for people to connect with you?

Hit me up on social media or email! I love to chat about celiac disease!

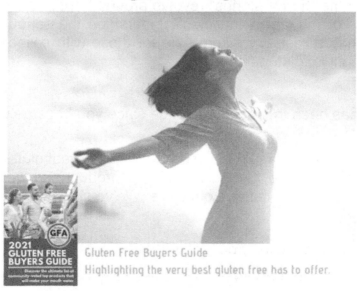

You know you are gluten free

Gluten Free Buyers Guide
Highlighting the very best gluten free has to offer.

When you hear the words
"dedicated fryer"

# Diana Duangnet

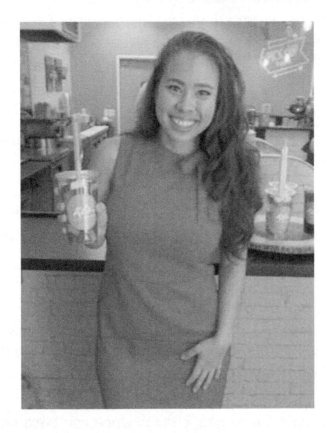

How long have you been gluten free?

I was diagnosed with Celiac disease 5 years ago.


Do you have any other dietary restrictions?

Luckily just gluten free!


What has been your biggest challenge thus far?

Traveling all the time for work (I'm a flight attendant) and pleasure and ensuring I always have something safe to eat.

Where is your favorite place to eat?

SO MANY PLACES! My top favorites include Modern Bread and Bagel (NYC), Honest Burgers (London), and Coquette's Bistro & Bakery (Colorado Springs).


Do you have any gluten related pet peeves?

When people don't know the difference between gluten free, dairy free, and vegan.


How has the Covid quarantine changed your diet habits?

Lots of home cooking and "traveling" around the world by trying out new recipes.


Do you have a gluten horror story?

While in Mississippi. "Hi, do you have anything gluten free?" "Oh honey, I don't know what gluten is, but we have the best fried chicken!"


What has been the biggest change since you became gluten free?

The initial learning curve was tough trying to navigate reading labels, cooking, and eating out at restaurants.


In ten years, a gluten free diet will be···

Understood and wildly accepted.


What is the best advice you received?

When in doubt, don't eat it.

What is the best way for people to connect with you?

You can check me out on

Instagram: @travelfarglutenfree

Facebook: www.facebook.com/travelfarglutenfree

YouTube: www.youtube.com/channel/UCmlxl-oGjmU5k5oks4cjBMA

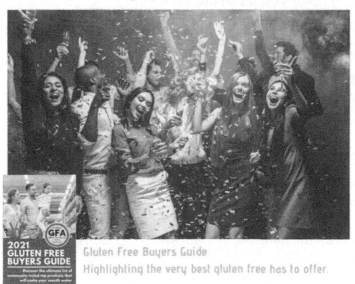

# Michael Frolichstein

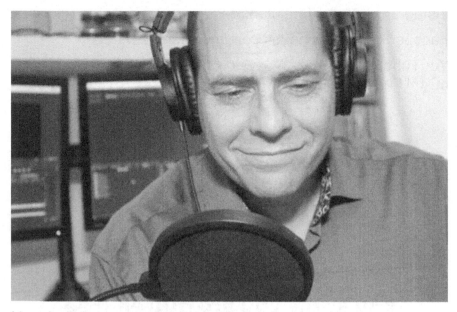

How long have you been gluten free?

11 years

Do you have any other dietary restrictions?

No

What has been your biggest challenge thus far?

Normally, my biggest challenge would be the social gatherings which include food, but during this time of social distancing, I'm finding that I am more anxious to order food from restaurants for take-out. I am wary of getting glutened.

Where is your favorite place to eat?

I have a few, but my favorite would be Wildfire. It is a classic steakhouse style restaurant with a full gluten free menu the size of their original, and excellent protocols in place so they consistently "do it right."  A nice touch is that they have our name in their system and just grab gluten free menus without us needing to ask. Plus, my wife and daughters love it, too!

Do you have any gluten related pet peeves?

My biggest pet peeve is that so many people can't wrap their minds around cross contamination.  I still get strange looks and eye rolls when avoiding gluten free foods in certain situations.  With The Celiac Project, I'm all about educating others, but sometimes in these personal situations I'm just frustrated and want to relax.

How has the Covid quarantine changed your diet habits?

Luckily, my wife, Ellen, is a great cook and is constantly making all of the favorite meals and treats that our family loves.  It has brought comfort during this time of uncertainty. Also, there have been many great guests on the podcast who have given us tips on how to have unique food experiences at home, which we are having fun experimenting with.

Do you have a gluten horror story?

Unfortunately, yes!  I guess we all have at least one, and when I tell this story around my kids, they just cringe.  We were making tacos and using a brand of tortillas that we thought at the time only made the corn variety.  Midway through dinner my daughter, Jessica, also a celiac, commented on the taste and texture being so amazing and different than what she was used to.  My wife and my eyes met in horror.  I ran to the kitchen, read the package and they were wheat tortillas. I was in total disbelief at the mistake and by then it was too late. I had one of the most terrible nights of my life.  So sick as a dog and I even passed out on the floor. It was the only time, to my knowledge, in the past 11 years that I knowingly consumed a gluten containing product.  It was a great reminder to always double and triple check the ingredients and make no assumptions.

What has been the biggest change since you became gluten free?

Since becoming gluten free 11 years ago, the level of daily brain fog, illness, and anxiety that permeated my life since childhood dissipated, and the renewed sense of how I could redefine myself moving forward was liberating.  Becoming gluten free changed more than my health, it changed the course of my life, inspiring me to start The Celiac Project-- my documentary and podcast, helping to raise awareness and bring our community together.  I am very grateful for that!

In ten years, a gluten free diet will be···

...not considered a fad.  My fear is that we might lose some products and restaurants, but the ones that remain will be more consistently trustworthy to the celiac and gluten intolerant community.  There is also a real possibility that in ten years there will be a treatment that will hopefully allow us to not worry about cross contamination, which would be a true game-changer.

What is the best advice you received?

Stay the course.  Although some people can feel better after just a couple of weeks on a gluten free diet, the majority of us take much longer to heal their gut and have their symptoms subside.  This takes patience, being good to yourself emotionally when you're having a tough time because getting better is not always a straight line.  Finding a good support system is also important so you don't feel alone.

What is the best way for people to connect with you?

If you would like to interact with me in a more personal way, go to www.celiacproject.com and join our Patreon #TCP Inner Circle where you can participate in a monthly live hangout with me, my podcast co-host, Cam Weiner, and our fellow community as we talk all things celiac and gluten free in an open, supportive, and positive forum. You can also email me at info@celiacproject.com and find me on Facebook, twitter or instagram @celiacproject

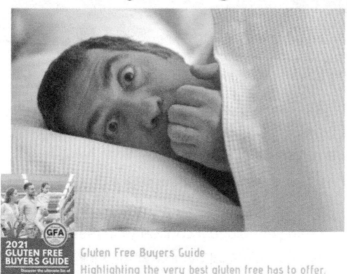

## You know you are gluten free

Gluten Free Buyers Guide
Highlighting the very best gluten free has to offer.

## When you have nightmares about eating regular food

# Cam Weiner

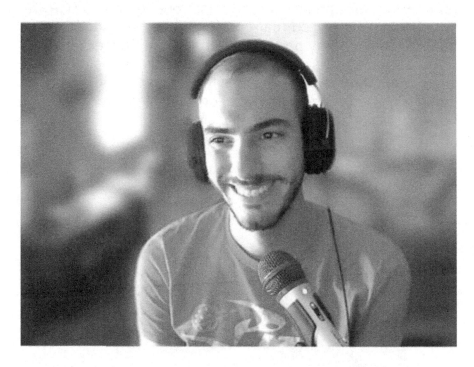

How long have you been gluten free?

7 years

Do you have any other dietary restrictions?

No nuts, soy, shellfish, or sesame either

What has been your biggest challenge thus far?

Balancing work and social events when sick with symptoms, or the added time for the diet (prep, travel, etc.). With enough time and planning, it is all possible though.

Where is your favorite place to eat?

Home!

Do you have any gluten related pet peeves?

The unclear separation between gluten-free and celiac safe.

How has the Covid quarantine changed your diet habits?

Not so much, no.

Do you have a gluten horror story?

Being undiagnosed was the real horror story haha. Since diagnosis though when getting contaminated I become prone to passing out and one time early on in my diagnosis I had a skateboard incident (very light I might say) that caused me to pass out two times in a row. Trying for a kickflip I hit my shin with the board and slowly got dizzy until I passed out. Since a much stricter gluten-free diet since then, I haven't had such incidents.

What has been the biggest change since you became gluten free?

I am less spontaneous and more cautious in dining/social situations, but I am also more thoughtful and sensitive to myself and other's needs now too.

In ten years, a gluten free diet will be···

Hopefully not needed. It will certainly be more normalized by then if it is still necessary.

What is the best advice you received?

It takes time to heal, be patient. Plan as much of your life as you would without thinking about the gluten-free part as possible and just make it work as best as you can.

What is the best way for people to connect with you?

Reach out to me at info@celiacproject.com or The Celiac Project on Facebook or Instagram

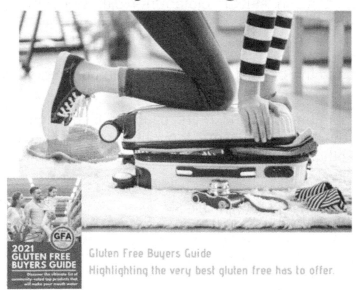

Gluten Free Buyers Guide
Highlighting the very best gluten free has to offer.

# Andrea Tucker

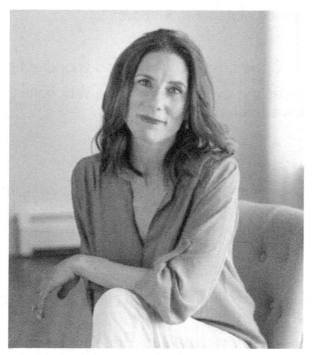

How long have you been gluten free?

10 years

Do you have any other dietary restrictions?

No

What has been your biggest challenge thus far?

Finding community and vetted sources of information. That was the motivation for starting my podcast, The Gluten Free News.

Where is your favorite place to eat?

HeartBeet Kitchen in Westmont, NJ

Do you have any gluten related pet peeves?

Products labeled gluten free that aren't.

How has the Covid quarantine changed your diet habits?

We are now eating every day at home with occasional take out from safe eateries.

Do you have a gluten horror story?

After many conversations at a small restaurant, my gluten free daughter found a piece of spaghetti in her salad. Needless to say, I let the manager know and have stayed far away from the establishment.

What has been the biggest change since you became gluten free?

The quality and quantity of gluten free products. The bread has gotten so much better too!

In ten years, a gluten free diet will be···

Well- understood and taken seriously.

What is the best advice you received?

To have a 504 plan for my daughter. It's an excellent tool for educating faculty and staff that follows her from year to year.

What is the best way for people to connect with you?

Social Media:

IG: baltimoreglutenfree FB: balimoreglutenfree Twitter: baltgf

# Emily Briand

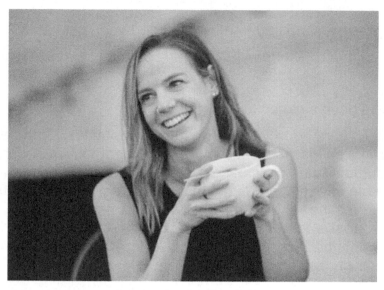

How long have you been gluten free?

13 years


Do you have any other dietary restrictions?

No


What has been your biggest challenge thus far?

The biggest challenge was finding safe, gluten free products 13 years ago. Now, there are so many incredible products and a ton of resources!


Where is your favorite place to eat?

My home! My husband and I love to cook together.


Do you have any gluten related pet peeves?

I wish the issue of cross contamination was more widely understood.

How has the Covid quarantine changed your diet habits?

Not too much. Though I have been baking a lot more treats.

Do you have a gluten horror story?

YES! 7 years ago I went to Bozeman, Montana. I had heard amazing things about the gluten free protocol at a certain restaurant. After confirming with the server 3 times that it was safe to eat, she brought my meal. Within a few minutes I started feeling very weird, when I asked her again she realized that she forgot to add any notes to the order and had put in for the regular dish. I had to leave immediately and was still charged for my meal!

What has been the biggest change since you became gluten free?

There are so many new and amazing products coming out!

In ten years, a gluten free diet will be⋯

Hopefully so much easier to navigate and avoid cross contamination.

What is the best advice you received?

Be your own advocate, no one knows your body like you do. It took me a while to feel confident declining food or products that I didn't feel safe eating.

What is the best way for people to connect with you?

Instagram. @im.emily.bean

# Kathlena, The Allergy Chef

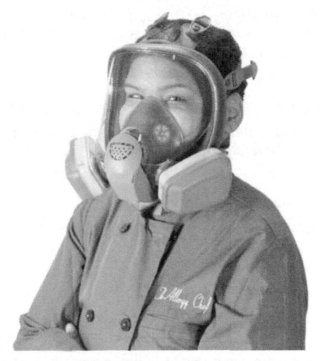

How long have you been gluten free?

10+ Years


Do you have any other dietary restrictions?

Over 200 food allergies and intolerances, some contact and airborne allergies, and can't drink most water.


What has been your biggest challenge thus far?

Getting companies to be completely transparent, even when asking all the "right/insider" questions.


Where is your favorite place to eat?

At home.

Do you have any gluten related pet peeves?

Lack of transparency for products certified gluten free that are made on shared equipment with wheat. That needs to be disclosed on the label.


How has the Covid quarantine changed your diet habits?

It hasn't. Our limitations always meant eating at home and that hasn't changed.


Do you have a gluten horror story?

A restaurant served us gluten free food that failed the Nima Sensor. Their peanut free drink also failed the Nima Peanut Sensor. Never went back.


What has been the biggest change since you became gluten free?

Learning all the unsavory industry practices that lead us to make more food on our own.


In ten years, a gluten free diet will be···

Hopefully cleaner with less consumer packaged goods that read like a science experiment.


What is the best advice you received?

Call companies.


What is the best way for people to connect with you?

TheAllergyChef.com has links to our membership site (RAISE), SF bakery, social media, and more.

# Audrey Roberts

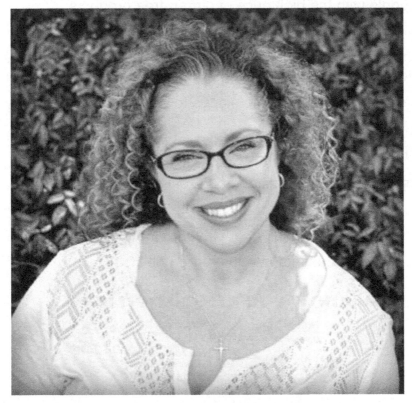

How long have you been gluten free?

11 years

Do you have any other dietary restrictions?

dairy-free

Where is your favorite place to eat?

I do not eat out much, but I enjoy Red Robin, PF Changs, Blaze Pizza, and Chick-fil-A. They are a few of the safe places I have been able to eat out at.

Do you have any gluten related pet peeves?

The price of gluten-free products. Most people and families struggle with the high price of gluten-free products.

What has been the biggest change since you became gluten free?

Traveling and having safe places to eat out.

In ten years, a gluten free diet will be···

Hopefully better understood and respected.

What is the best way for people to connect with you?

https://www.mamaknowsglutenfree.com/

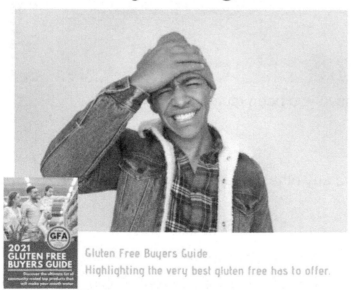

**You know you are gluten free**

Gluten Free Buyers Guide
Highlighting the very best gluten free has to offer.

**When you blow your paycheck at the grocery store**

# Gluten Free Product Registration

By submitting your products into The Gluten Free Awards (GFA), you are automatically entering products into the Annual Gluten Free Buyers Guide. There are only 10 slots available in each category and we limit brands to 3 submissions per category. If you are a marketer representing multiple brands, this typically will not apply. Slots can fill quickly so we recommend submitting your registration ASAP. The absolute deadline for registration is August 22nd however, we cannot guarantee you that the category is already full.

## "How do I get into the Gluten Free Awards?"

How it works:

1. Fill out the registration form by adding the quantities and product names.

(A free half page ad is given for every 5 products or full-page ad for 10 products.)

2. If wanted, add additional ad space to registration.

3. Email the registration form to Jayme@GlutenFreeBuyersGuide.com

4. We will follow up with a confirmation and invoice.

If you have any questions call customer support at 828-455-9734

**"Wait, I have tons of questions still"**

## Most common questions:

### Q: I am having a hard time understanding how to submit or products.

A: Using this Registration Form will help. If lost, don't hesitate to call or email. 828-455-9734

## Q: What are the image specs you need?

A: Our graphic team just needs images that are PDF, JPEG or PNG at 300 dpi or greater. The team will normally resize images based on the publishing media. Normally the product pictures and descriptions from your website will work just fine.

Full Page Ad Size 384 by 576 px

Half Page Ad Size 384 by 288 px

## Q: Is there a word count for product descriptions?

A: No, we normally don't use product descriptions just product names and images.

## Q: If we submit 10 products do we get 1 free full-page ad and 2 free half page ads?

A: Sorry, please choose one or the other. You can always purchase additional ad space.

## Q: Can we run a full-page ad without entering the awards program?

A: Yes.

## Q: Do we need to send you product samples?

A: No. The gluten-free community votes for your products.

## Q: Will we be in the guide if we don't win an award?

A: Yes, all products submitted will be visible as nominees.

## Q: Can we use the GFA Nominee and Winner Badge on our product packaging, website and other related media?

A: Yes, we highly recommend using the badges to differentiate your products from the rest. If you happen to need higher resolution images don't hesitate to ask. Read our media terms here.

**Need to talk about your order or have questions? Give us a call.**

828-455-9734

or email

Josh@GlutenFreeBuyersGuide.com

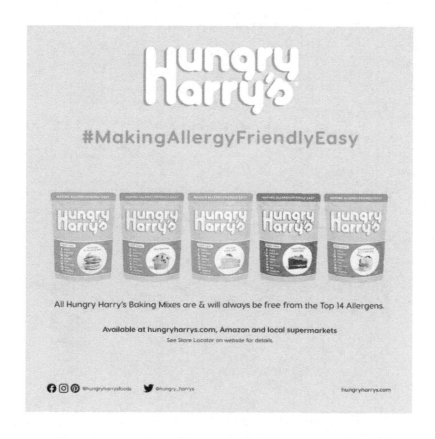

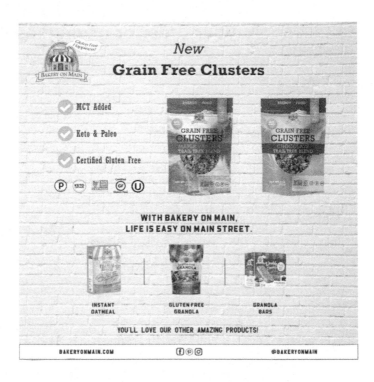

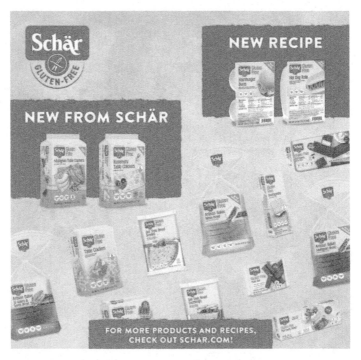

# From our family to yours, have a happy and healthy gluten free lifestyle.

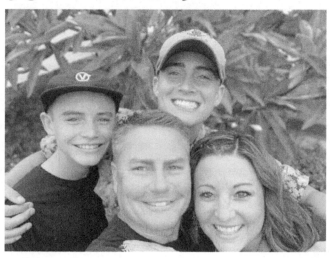

## The Schieffer Family

Josh (Dad with Celiac) Chief Marketing Officer

Jayme (Mom) VP Operations

Blake (20)

Jacob (16 Celiac)

Keep up to date with us, the awards, and future buyer guides at GlutenFreeBuyersGuide.com

**Notes:**

## COMING SOON - REGISTER NOW

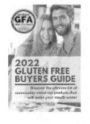 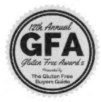

# 12TH ANNUAL
# GLUTEN FREE
# AWARDS HOSTED BY

THE GLUTEN FREE BUYERS GUIDE